THE ART OF DEMENTIA CARE

Jane Verity & Daniel Kuhn

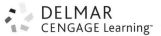

DELMAR
CENGAGE Learning™

Australia • Brazil • Japan • Korea • Mexico • Singapore • Spain • United Kingdom • United States

DELMAR
CENGAGE Learning™

The Art of Dementia Care
Jane Verity, Daniel Kuhn

Vice President, Health Care
  Business Unit:
  William Brottmiller

Director of Learning
  Solutions: Matthew Kane

Managing Editor:
  Marah Bellegarde

Acquisitions Editor:
  Matthew Seeley

Editorial Assistant:
  Megan Tarquinio

Marketing Director:
  Jennifer McAvey

Marketing Manager:
  Michele McTighe

Marketing Coordinator:
  Chelsey Iaquinta

Production Director:
  Carolyn Miller

Content Project Manager:
  Anne Sherman

Art Director: Jack Pendleton

For product information and technology assistance, contact us at **Cengage Learning Customer & Sales Support, 1-800-354-9706**

For permission to use material from this text or product, submit all requests online at **www.cengage.com/permissions** Further permissions questions can be emailed to **permissionrequest@cengage.com**

Library of Congress Control Number: 2007018127

ISBN-13: 978-1-4018-9951-6

ISBN-10: 1-4018-9951-X

Delmar
Executive Woods
5 Maxwell Drive
Clifton Park, NY 12065
USA

Cengage Learning is a leading provider of customized learning solutions with office locations around the globe, including Singapore, the United Kingdom, Australia, Mexico, Brazil, and Japan. Locate your local office at **www.cengage.com/global**

Cengage Learning products are represented in Canada by Nelson Education, Ltd.

To learn more about Delmar, visit **www.cengage.com/delmar**

Purchase any of our products at your local bookstore or at our preferred online store **www.ichapters.com**

Notice to the Reader

Printed in the United States of America
4 5 6 7 11 10 09

616.83
V517

CONTENTS

A C K N O W L E D G M E N T S

Grateful acknowledgment is first given to the late Dr. Tom Kitwood, as well as Dr. Murna Downs, Dr. Dawn Brooker, and other members of the Bradford Dementia Group at the University of Bradford in England for their pioneering work in advocating for the health and well-being of people with dementia. Dr. Kitwood's person-centered approach to dementia care was described in his 1997 book, *Dementia Reconsidered: The Person Comes First.* Kind permission to use some of his concepts, known as "personal detractors," has been granted by the book's publisher, Open University Press.

Thanks also to Dr. Konrad Maurer of the Department of Psychiatry, University of Frankfurt on Main for allowing the use of the photo of Auguste Deiter, the person first described by Dr. Alois Alzheimer with the disease that bears his name.

Chris Bell of Dementia Care Australia is gratefully acknowledged for her editorial assistance. Marah Bellegarde and other members of the publishing team at Delmar Learning are also owed a debt of gratitude for their encouragement and assistance.

ABOUT THE AUTHORS

Jane Verity   Originally from Denmark and now living in Australia, Jane is the founder and director of Dementia Care Australia (www.dementiacareaustralia.com), an independent information and education organization that aims to change society's attitude toward dementia and show that improvement is achievable. Her philosophy is that it is possible to rekindle the spark of life in people with dementia and in those who care for them. She has developed the internationally acclaimed *Spark of Life* program designed to improve the well-being of people with dementia.

Jane is a qualified occupational and family therapist, with more than 25 years of international experience. She is a master practitioner in neuro-linguistic programming and one of few people in this field who applies this communication process to all aspects of dementia. She has recently been appointed Eden Alternative Mentor for the entire Scandinavian community. Jane is also a professional speaker and holds the highest accreditation (CSP) of the National Speakers Association. She speaks regularly at international conferences and consults with both government and private sectors.

Jane has authored multiple publications and articles, including the *Spark of Life* newsletter and her first Danish title, *Demens—Lær at genantæde Livsgnisten (Dementia—Learn to Rekindle the Spark of Life)* was published by Forlaget Munksgaard Danmark A/S in 2005.

Jane understands the frustrations and joys of caring for someone with dementia at a professional as well as a personal level. Her own mother lived with dementia for over 10 years before she passed away in 2005.

Daniel Kuhn   A native of Chicago, where he still resides, Dan has worked in various settings within the fields of health care and aging for more than 30 years. He received a master's degree in social work from the University of Illinois at Chicago and is a licensed clinical social worker. Since 1987 he has focused primarily on the care of individuals and families affected by Alzheimer's disease and related dementias. Dan is currently the director of the Professional Training Institute for the Alzheimer's Association—Greater Illinois Chapter. Previously, he was director of education at Mather LifeWays Institute on Aging and director of education at the Rush Alzheimer's Disease Center.

Dan has authored or co-authored more than forty publications, including the popular guidebook *Alzheimer's Early Stages: First Steps for Family, Friends and Caregivers* (Hunter House Publishers, 2nd edition, 2003). He has been involved in developing several award-winning online training programs and educational videos, including *A Thousand Tomorrows: Intimacy, Sexuality and Alzheimer's Disease* by Terra Nova Films. He is a past board member of the American Society on Aging and currently serves on the editorial boards of several peer-reviewed journals.

Dan has been privileged to know thousands of individuals and families who have courageously faced dementia and countless professionals who care deeply about them. His grandfather died of dementia in a nursing home after many years of home care.

FOREWORD

THE ART OF GOOD DEMENTIA CARE

Jane Verity and Dan Kuhn are fabulous advocates for people living with dementia in residential care homes everywhere. Many books on care appear to be written by people who have never considered what the human experience of dementia feels like. Through the eyes of three people with dementia, Earl, Mildred, and Lucinda, this book clearly describes the challenges that this experience brings. It also describes the joy that people with dementia can experience when those around them truly meet their needs.

Jane and Dan are also fine advocates for people who spend their days and nights at work caring for those living in care homes. The world of care work is often characterized by dullness and apathy and those who do this work are seen as being in low-status jobs. Within the pages of this book, we learn that this does not need to be the reality. Jane and Dan describe the skills needed by direct care workers as those of a great artist. Their words and ideas exude optimism and energy as they describe the way in which care workers can make a real difference in the lives of people with dementia.

Although this book is designed to be relevant for direct care staff, there is much within its pages that will appeal to a far broader audience. Administrators, managers, owners, and board members of care facilities, as well as professional practitioners, government officials, and educators will find much here that will help them support the work of those delivering direct care. It is a practical book, written with great humanity that has the ability to change hearts and minds.

Much of this book builds on ideas from the late Dr. Tom Kitwood, who was my mentor and friend. He would have been proud of this book. It puts people being cared for at the center of the stage and gives us a better insight into the world that they see. It is full of hope for all of us.

Professor Dawn Brooker
Bradford Dementia Group
University of Bradford
United Kingdom

INTRODUCTION

The underlying belief behind this book is that every human being has the capacity for growth if given the opportunity. This is true for you as a professional caregiver, as well as for people with dementia. This book provides insights into their special needs. In particular, it will show how your approach can enable them to become contented, happy, and full of joy. You can learn to experience meaningful connections with them on a daily basis. *The Art of Dementia Care* is intended to serve your professional interests and the interests of residents in your care.

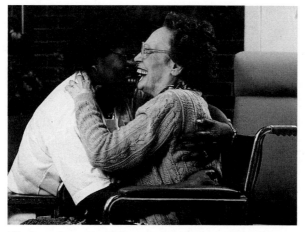

The joy of meaningful connection between friends.

It is also our belief that the sum of small acts of genuine empathy, encouragement, love, and fun can improve the lives of people with dementia. *You* can and do make a positive difference in the lives of your residents. When this happens, you will also make a positive difference in your own life by becoming a more caring and complete individual.

We liken this work to being an artist. It takes creativity, patience, and skill to achieve positive results. Just like the painter, sculptor, or architect, you already have certain skills that you have acquired with education, training, and experience. The more you learn and develop your skills, the more rewarding the results will be. This book will give you fresh ideas and new skills that can be put into practice immediately.

OUR GOALS

Our overall purpose in writing this book is to offer an easy-to-read, practical, and helpful guide for all those who provide support, encouragement, and care for people with dementia in formal care settings, such as nursing homes, assisted living facilities, and other residential care situations. Regardless of your education, training, or experience, if you are directly involved in the care of people with dementia, this book is intended for you. We hope it will be read by nursing assistants, personal care workers, activity staff, dietary aides, nurses, social workers, therapists, and others who do the day-to-day work in residential care settings.

Quite simply, we want you to be able to provide not just good dementia care, but great dementia care. We wish to inspire you with the possibilities that lie within your power to create a personally rewarding career. We have set out to achieve three main goals:

1. To introduce you to the idea that caring for people with dementia is a work of art;
2. To introduce a shift in focus from a medical model of care to a relationship model of care;

3. To honor and empower you, the artist, in the same way we encourage you to honor and empower those in your care.

In this book, we do not attempt to cover all aspects of dementia or dementia care. Such books already exist and some of our favorites are listed in the final section, Selected References and Resources. It is our intention here to help you experience, see, hear, and feel that success is the result of *subtle* changes in your thinking and behavior. As an artist, you are the most important asset you bring into the lives of people with dementia. This book represents a shift:

- from defining dementia as a medical problem to defining it as a social and psychological challenge for those experiencing dementia;
- from focusing on what's "wrong" with the person with dementia to building on their strengths and resources;
- from focusing on difficult behavior as a symptom of dementia to an expression of unmet needs;
- from focusing on the physical needs of the person with dementia to also meeting other human needs, such as social, emotional, psychological, and spiritual;
- from focusing on families as mere visitors to people in need of healing and care.

We will use examples from everyday care situations. Some examples represent pleasant experiences that enhance the quality of life. Other examples represent unpleasant experiences that diminish the quality of life.

Becoming an artist of dementia care is not easy. It involves challenging yet important human work. Not everyone can handle its demands. We encourage you to look deep inside yourself to see if you have what it takes. You may not have the personality, maturity, skills, or interests suited to meet the special needs of people with dementia. You may need to ask yourself if you are in the right field.

You deserve to enjoy your work and be the best that you can be. If you have what it takes to be an artist of dementia care, you and those in your care will be richly rewarded.

THE LAYOUT

The six chapters of this book will prompt you to rethink your attitudes and behaviors toward people with dementia. We will explain some outdated attitudes toward people with dementia and reveal new insights into their need for individualized approaches. In Chapter 1, we tell the story of Dr. Alzheimer and how we must build a bridge to reach into the world of people with dementia. In Chapter 2, we describe what it means to be an artist of dementia care. Chapter 3 highlights the need to shift from a medical model of care to a relationship model of care. In Chapter 4, we explain challenging behaviors associated with dementia as expressions of unmet needs. Chapter 5 explains ways to support families as they cope with the losses associated with a loved one's dementia. Finally, Chapter 6 encourages you to become a great artist by practicing what we call "uplifts"—daily occasions for connecting with your residents in ways that bring them joy.

THREE STAGES OF DEMENTIA

There have been many descriptions written about different stages of dementia, but here we refer to just three stages: early, middle, and late. These stages often fluctuate and overlap. They focus on symptoms in general terms and do not explain how people respond differently to their particular symptoms. Stages and symptoms don't do justice to the uniqueness of each person with dementia. However, an understanding of the different stages is useful to identify and meet the needs of each person at a particular time. In this book, we use the names of three people to highlight the differences among the three stages of dementia. You may wish to substitute these three names with those of people you know.

- Early stage: **Earl**
- Middle stage: **Mildred**
- Late stage: **Lucinda**

Early Stage: Earl

People in the early stage of dementia usually communicate clearly using words and sentences the same way most people do. They are, however, more forgetful than usual; for example they may not remember events or might misplace things. Their thinking skills become diminished as shown by difficulty in solving problems that would have been easy in the past. They may have trouble finding the right word or recalling the name of a person, place, or thing. Those around them start to question or comment on the changes in them. In turn, they may feel embarrassed or frightened when they recognize changes in their memory or thinking. They are likely to be creative in avoiding this painful reality such as refusing to join a social

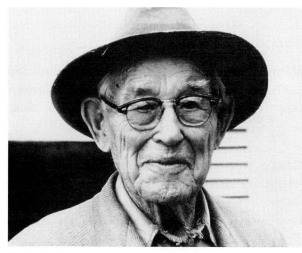

Earl who is in the early stage of dementia.

activity for fear of forgetting the names of friends. Generally, people in the early stage of dementia may:

- Repeat the same questions, such as when Earl asks what day or what time the next meal is to be served.
- Compensate for memory loss, such as when Earl makes up a story to fill in the missing details; he is not lying, but trying to maintain a façade.
- Blame others for their memory lapses, such as when Earl accuses someone of taking his glasses when he cannot find them.
- Express anger or irritation in response to direct questions requiring memory or thinking skills, such as when Earl is asked what year he was born and he replies angrily, "That is none of your business!"
- Offer creative responses to embarrassing situations, such as when Earl's glasses are found among his underwear and he explains, "They must have found a new home!"
- Try to exercise control over a situation, such as when Earl decides that a certain chair in the lounge belongs to him and he yells at others for sitting in "his" chair.

Middle Stage: Mildred

People in the middle stage of dementia are more forgetful about recent events, become easily confused, and have difficulty finding or using the right words. They increasingly need help from others. People in the middle stage generally may:

- Compensate for trouble with words, such as when Mildred says "rain stick" instead of umbrella or substitutes "sugar" for salt.
- Lose the initiative to start and continue an activity, such as when Mildred sits and stares at a game, which is right in front of her.

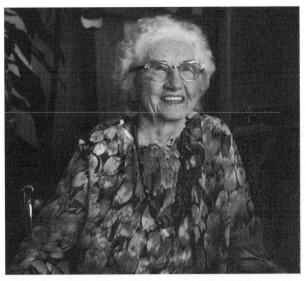

Mildred who is in the middle stage of dementia.

- Get confused about the intentions of others, such as when Mildred becomes agitated while being assisted with a bath.
- Become disoriented in regard to place, such as when Mildred cannot find her own room.
- Begin to mix up the generations, such as when Mildred misidentifies her own daughter as her sister or believes that her deceased mother is still alive.
- Lose the ability to handle some personal care tasks, such as when Mildred is unable to bathe on her own.

Late Stage: Lucinda

The symptoms of dementia are quite pronounced in the late stage. The need for support from others for completing the most basic daily activities is commonplace. People in the late stage of dementia generally may:

- Communicate through body language, sounds, and actions instead of words and sentences, such as when Lucinda

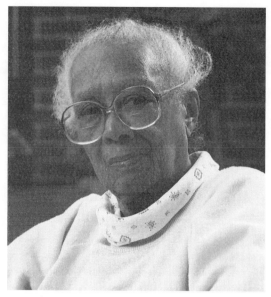

Lucinda who is in the late stage of dementia.

motions with her hands that she no longer wants to eat her food.

- Live in a personal world, such as when Lucinda reorganizes the chairs in the dining room to relive a time when she was in charge of the dining room of her own home.
- Use objects or body parts to fulfill emotional needs, such as when Lucinda clutches her doll or kneads imaginary dough.
- Walk around to prevent boredom or to look for someone or something, such as when Lucinda paces the corridor to keep herself busy.
- Quietly observe the activity and emotions of others, such as when Lucinda watches other residents and staff without becoming engaged with them.
- Need support with most or all of her personal care activities, such as when Lucinda needs assistance to use the bathroom.

OUR WISH FOR YOU

We must continuously practice the art of dementia care in order to achieve the best possible results. It is our hope that this book will enable you to identify yourself as an artist and improve your skills. People with dementia will benefit from what you learn and put into practice. Their families will benefit too. *You* are the best asset they have right now. It is indeed an awesome responsibility to imagine that you hold the key to the quality of someone else's life. It is our sincere hope that you will take satisfaction in becoming a great artist of dementia care and giving your residents the best quality of life possible in their time of need.

1

DR. ALZHEIMER AND
AUGUSTE DEITER

"Just as despair can come to one only from other human beings, hope, too, can be given to one only by other human beings."

—Elie Weisel,
Nobel Peace Prize winner

In 1906, a physician named Alois Alzheimer reported to a group of fellow doctors in Germany about a patient he had cared for; a woman by the name of Auguste Deiter. She had been brought into a mental hospital in Frankfurt, Germany, because she could no longer remember her husband, her children, and other familiar people and places. She needed attention that her family could no longer provide, and she spent the last few years of her life in this facility under the supervision of Dr. Alzheimer.

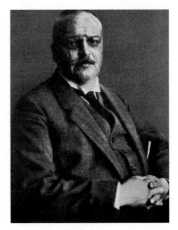

Dr. Alois Alzheimer

According to Dr. Alzheimer's notes, Auguste was unable to respond accurately to questions about either her past or present situation. She was disoriented and had difficulty finding words. Although her arms and legs worked well, she could no longer do simple things like dressing and bathing herself. Her language, behavior, and emotions appeared strange. Over time, her problems with memory and thinking grew worse until she needed help with everything. Finally, Auguste became bedridden and died from pneumonia. Dr. Alzheimer guessed from the start that something was wrong with her brain. He described her symptoms in terms of what was to become known as dementia.

After Auguste died, Dr. Alzheimer examined her brain under a microscope. He observed that the brain had shrunk from its normal size. He also described tiny abnormalities he referred to as "tangles" and "plaques" that he thought were signs that cells in the brain had died for mysterious reasons. The symptoms experienced by Auguste eventually became known as dementia of the Alzheimer's type, or Alzheimer's disease.

Today, one hundred years later, scientists are still puzzled about how dementia develops in the brain. Until the causes are known, it is difficult to invent effective medical treatments, cures, or means of prevention. At best, the few drugs available now to treat dementia have modest benefits and do not stop its progression. However, the good news is that *you,* as the caregiver, possess the knowledge, ingenuity, and skills to promote a good quality of life for people with dementia. Despite their limits in thinking, remembering, and doing for themselves, you can help compensate for their difficulties and enable them to use their remaining abilities. Your efforts may offer far more benefits than any drugs could.

A LOST SELF

To gain some insight into how you can make life better for people like Auguste Deiter, let us take a further look into her situation. It is fair to assume that conditions in a long-term care facility in Germany a century ago were poor by modern standards. Things we take for granted today, such as plumbing and electricity, were not yet commonplace, making life unpleasant for residents and staff alike. Dozens of residents were placed together in large, cold rooms. They probably had little or nothing to do to occupy their time. Staff kept them fed, clean, clothed, and housed but little else was done for them.

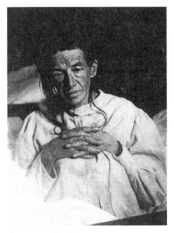

Auguste Deiter

It can also be assumed that the residents were treated as if they were "crazy." No one knew what to do to make their lives enjoyable. They were no longer rational. They did not fit into the "normal" world and were separated from society for their own safety. Their lives as they had known them were finished. In truth, they were no longer living but waiting to die. It is difficult to imagine how awful life must have been for Auguste and the other residents living in that facility a century ago.

Dr. Alzheimer provided a glimpse into the poor quality of life through his written description about Auguste. He asked her questions that she could not answer. He asked her to perform tasks that she could no longer do. Auguste may have wondered, "Doesn't he realize that I can no longer remember and think the way I used to? Why doesn't he know my limits and help me succeed at something for a change? Why is he pestering me with stupid questions? Doesn't he know that I am still a person and need self-respect, dignity, and love? Why don't the people here understand my broken language and thoughts? I am doing the best I can, but they are making my life harder by trying to get me to act 'normal.' Can't they accommodate me instead of insisting that I fit into their world?"

According to Dr. Alzheimer's notes, Auguste repeatedly remarked, "I have lost myself." This is a sad yet not surprising comment by someone removed from her home, her family, her friends, and familiar way of life, and then put into a place filled with strangers. Nothing about this facility resembled home and no one reminded her of anyone in her past. With little or nothing to do, except eat and sleep, she probably felt like there was no purpose or meaning in her life. Auguste must have felt very lonely and fearful. No one bothered to help her find herself again. No one understood her plea for help or saw life through her eyes.

LESSONS LEARNED

We can look back a century ago and hope that staff then did their best with what they knew at the time. Lack of knowledge and other resources stood in the way of offering their residents a good life. We like to think that care of people like Auguste Deiter, as well as their environment, have improved nowadays. Today, countless government regulations exist to protect frail people from neglect or mistreatment. Strict standards about staff training and quality of care also exist so that people with dementia are generally treated better now.

And yet, today, we hear different versions of Auguste's cry for help when people with dementia say things like, "Help me! Help me! Where am I? I want to go home. Can you help me? What am I supposed to do here?" Sometimes they lack the words to express how they feel and act out their emotional suffering by screaming or striking out at others. Some people with dementia give up trying after a while. They may sit passively or sleep much of the time. If you listen carefully to their words or interpret their behavior, perhaps you can hear the echo of Auguste's troubling words, "I have lost myself."

The fact is that Dr. Alzheimer and his staff might have been able to help Auguste find herself, but they treated her difficulties as medical symptoms beyond their capacity to understand or cure. Perhaps they assumed that she was "too far gone" and did not know how to reach her. They may have believed that not much could be done. After all, she no longer acted, spoke, or thought in normal ways—so why bother? *They did not step into* **her** *world and she was left to struggle in* **their** *world.* They did not take responsibility for making her life better. They concluded that nothing could be done to improve it.

When you first began working with people with dementia, what were your first impressions? Did you believe that little could be done for them except to keep them clean and fed? Did you think that they were beyond all understanding? How have your attitudes changed as you have become more experienced? Can you see the difference you make in the lives of people in your care? How do you measure success?

TAKING RESPONSIBILITY

Imagine for a moment that you are suddenly transported to a foreign country. You are completely unprepared for this strange trip. You do not know the language, customs, or the people. You have no food or money. You are without a road map and you do not know your final destination. You wonder, "What am I doing here?" This must be a bad dream—except you cannot wake up. People who talk to you don't make any sense. When you try to speak to them, they give you strange looks. You do not fit into this place. You are like the proverbial fish out of water—outside your comfort zone. You feel utterly alone and frightened.

Finally, a woman approaches you who can see that you are in trouble. She speaks a few words of your language and uses gestures to help you feel at ease. She offers you her hand and says that she will lead you to a safe place. Your fears and worries are slowly replaced by calm. You cannot buy or cook food, so she helps you to eat and drink. She constantly reaches out to find ways of connecting with you. She puts herself in your shoes and anticipates your needs. She does what you cannot do for yourself. She enables you to use whatever skills you have in order to be as self-sufficient as possible. Instead of treating you like a stranger, she accepts you as a friend. Gradually, you begin to feel good about yourself again. You slowly gain confidence in finding your way through this foreign land. You know that, if faced with trouble again, your new friend will help you. Life is good again after all.

In the situation described above, your nightmare had a happy ending. Why? Because of another person's genuine care and concern for you. Someone was willing to serve as a bridge into your world and help you feel at peace. As you may have guessed, people with dementia often feel like the stranger who is lost and alone. You can become a bridge builder—the one who makes a good life possible for them.

Compared to a century ago, we now possess a better understanding of dementia and dementia care. It is generally accepted that people with dementia deserve more than physical care. All aspects of their well-being should be addressed: mind, body, and spirit. They can enjoy life despite their impairments. You can learn ways to reach out to and connect with them so they feel good about themselves. In doing so, you can feel good about making a positive difference in their lives.

A FRESH APPROACH

In the late 1980s, Dr. Tom Kitwood, founder of the Bradford Dementia Research Group in England, developed a fresh approach that challenged the traditional way of thinking about dementia and dementia care. He called his approach *person-centered care*. The focus of this care is on the individual person with dementia rather than on the disease or its symptoms. In spite of the limits of drugs used to treat dementia, Dr. Kitwood offered the encouraging news that much could be done with human ingenuity, knowledge, and skills to lessen the effects of dementia.

Dr. Kitwood understood that the physical damage to an individual's brain caused by dementia did not fully explain the effects on the person. He had observed that the manner in which people with dementia were cared for contributed greatly to their experience. In this way, he discovered that dementia was not just a medical problem, but also a social and psychological one. He also observed that many of the problems experienced by people with dementia were due to poor communication by their caregivers. On the other hand, Dr. Kitwood discovered that skillful and compassionate listeners could lessen the effects of dementia through good communication. Furthermore, people with dementia could actually thrive in the midst of a supportive and encouraging community. A person-centered approach could make this a daily reality for everyone with dementia.

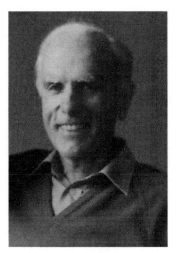

Dr. Tom Kitwood

So what is person-centered care? More than a philosophy, it is a way of thinking and doing on behalf of people who have dementia with the goal of promoting their overall well-being. Person-centered care has several major elements that you can learn and share with others.

Understanding the Individual's Perspective

First and foremost, person-centered care requires you to look at the world from the perspective of the individual person with dementia. In this view, his or her experience is accepted as reality. This reality helps to explain the behavior of the person with dementia. No matter how strange a behavior may appear to you, it makes sense and has personal meaning to the one with dementia. The key challenge is to put yourself "in the shoes" of the individual in order to understand how he or she is thinking, feeling, or experiencing the world. You look for signs of their discomfort, fear, worry, or loneliness and take active steps to prevent or minimize these negative feelings. You also watch for signs of pleasure, comfort, and joy and take active steps to increase these positive feelings.

In short, you make it your business to be a second set of eyes and ears for them. This becomes your personal mission. You can then better respond to the kind of help and support that each person needs. In doing so, you can restore the person's self-confidence and self-esteem, which are often threatened by dementia symptoms.

Valuing People with Dementia

The second major part of the person-centered approach is about valuing people with dementia. At first glance, you may think that it is obvious that they are people worthy of respect as full human beings. However, society places a high value on thinking, memory, and productivity. Strong biases exist against disabled people, especially older people with dementia who no longer contribute to society in the usual ways. They are easily disregarded because often they cannot speak for themselves.

A person-centered approach acknowledges the special contributions that people with dementia can still offer at an emotional and spiritual level. It considers that everyone deserves to be treated with respect in the same manner we would expect to be treated. Dementia is no reason to be treated as a second-class citizen. A person-centered approach ensures that the dignity of each person is upheld.

A Whole Person Approach

The person-centered approach also emphasizes that people with dementia must be seen and treated as whole persons. After all, they lived for many decades before the onset of their problems with memory and thinking. Each person's life must be seen in its entirety, and not just at this particular time when one's needs and impairments are so evident. By seeing people first and dementia second, you see possibilities instead of only problems. You see opportunities to engage them in using their remaining abilities. You work to help them discover ways to live life to the fullest, in spite of the dementia. You appreciate who they have been in the past, who they are now, and who they can still become.

Your work requires high levels of ability, creativity, and insight. You can make good things happen for them every day and with every encounter. They rely on you to bring out the best in them—something they can no longer do easily for themselves.

A SET OF BELIEFS

In order to practice the art of dementia care, mistaken ideas that people with dementia are crazy, worthless, and beyond hope must be challenged. To some degree, most of us harbor such biases or stereotypes that cast people with dementia in a bad light. We need to change these negative and undermining beliefs, which indirectly influence our entire attitude. A positive approach to dementia involves adopting five beliefs and implementing these in our daily work. In doing so, you can change the lives of people with dementia for the better. You will also find your work more rewarding than you ever imagined.

Belief #1: A positive social environment can minimize the disabling effects of dementia.

The circumstances or conditions that surround us are referred to as our *environment.* An environment is not limited to physical circumstances or conditions. The behaviors and emotions of people also influence the environment. Every personal encounter you have with people who have dementia may affect their social and psychological environment. Your actions and attitudes influence whether they experience ill-being or well-being. *Your feelings are contagious—people with dementia "catch" your attitude and mood.* A good relationship with you can create a positive environment for them, while a poor relationship can break their spirit.

A helpful and supportive relationship enables them to use their remaining abilities, just as a cane or walker can aid someone with mobility problems. Drugs and technology cannot satisfy one's social and emotional needs. Only people can satisfy these human needs.

A reassuring hug or a big smile may offset the disabling effects of dementia. There is no substitute for the power of a good relationship between you and your residents. The quality of their lives relies in great measure on the quality of love and care you share with them.

Quality of life for those in care depends largely on the quality of their relationships. Their world is slowly shrinking. They progressively lose their abilities to navigate their own way and to meet their own needs. Choices become limited and others, like you, take over many decisions for them. Dr. Bill Thomas, founder of the Eden Alternative, a movement to radically change the culture of long-term care facilities, says that you can become a "world maker" for those in your care. This is an awesome responsibility. You have the power to make their world miserable or enjoyable. You are in a unique position to offer them many simple gifts, such as a gentle touch, a warm smile, or a pleasant voice. You can help create moments of closeness and enjoyment for them. You have the power and the privilege to remind them that they still deserve life's pleasures.

Belief #2: People with dementia are individuals with unique personalities, backgrounds, and preferences.

Every person with dementia has a unique history that spans many decades. Each one has a life story filled with many interesting chapters. Experiences from the past helped shape the person you see today. Discovering how people lived before you met them can be very useful. You may be surprised to learn who was a teacher, a musician, a banker, or a football player. You may gain insight into their current behavior and feelings by learning about their past roles as siblings, parents, grandparents, or great-grandparents.

You may be able to tap into their long-term memory and help them talk about their personal stories. You can often bring their old memories to life again.

People with dementia are individuals who deserve to be treated in personalized ways. Some may be naturally quiet and others may be outspoken. Some people are picky about food while others eat

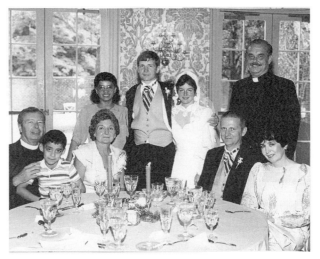

Photos serve as windows to our past.

almost anything. Some like bingo; others don't. Some are physically attractive; others may possess mainly inner beauty. It should not be assumed that everyone enjoys the same things or shares the same tastes. Individual preferences need to be taken into account to suit each person's unique needs. Each person is special.

Belief #3: People with dementia thrive in the midst of fun-loving relationships with adults, children, and pets.

People with dementia tend to focus on the present. They might dwell upon the past and rarely talk about the future. For the most part, living in the moment becomes a way of life. The quality of the relationships they are experiencing right now is of the utmost importance. Fun-loving relationships not only enable them to survive the disabling effects of their dementia, but they also help them to thrive.

You can teach others how to help people with dementia to thrive. Just talking about it is not enough. You have to show others how to have a fun-loving relationship with them. Young children are experts at it. They are free from inhibitions and accept others without judgment. People with dementia naturally show affection in response to loving people and pets.

You have seen people with dementia express delight when chatting with a friend, looking at a picture, singing a song, playing with a child, dancing a waltz, smelling a flower, or reciting a prayer. You have seen them give thanks with a word or a smile. You have seen them act kindly toward others. These good experiences are made possible because others, like you, fostered a positive relationship with them. You created the conditions necessary for such enjoyment. Anyone who is understanding and compassionate can make a contribution.

Belief #4: People with dementia are entitled to achieve their maximum potential in body, mind, and spirit.

Dementia should not serve as an excuse for low expectations about the abilities of people with dementia. They may appear disinterested in the world around them, but they are still capable of enjoyment if given the right opportunities. They deserve to be able to achieve their maximum potential and experience positive well-being on a daily basis.

This means that you must take active steps to compensate for their disabilities. In the same manner that those with mobility problems are offered rehabilitation or aids such as walkers or canes, people with dementia deserve the best possible effort to restore lost functions. For example, someone who has stopped eating independently should not be assumed to have lost that ability permanently. You do your best to help restore that lost skill. Just because someone has stopped talking does not mean that all understanding has been lost. You still communicate with words but may have to learn better ways to communicate non-verbally. For example, someone with language problems may enjoy self-expression through singing, dancing, painting, or drawing.

Efforts to restore abilities should always be a goal. If this goal is no longer realistic, you can help minimize their disabilities. Be open to possibilities instead of limits. This belief will shape your thinking and your actions.

Belief #5: People with dementia have something valuable to teach all of us.

If you stop to think about it, people with dementia serve as living reminders about important human values. They teach us that there is more to life than being productive through physical work or intellectual pursuits. They teach us about living in the moment instead of worrying about the past or the future. Their slowed way of thinking and doing contrasts sharply with the rapid pace of our modern lifestyle. They teach us about communicating without words due to their diminished language skills.

The majority of older people do not die suddenly, but, rather, develop a chronic condition that results in physical or mental disabilities. People with such frailties remind all of us that our bodies and minds may not always be healthy. People with dementia teach us that the physical and mental aspects of ourselves may slowly fade away. Their presence forces us to consider the spiritual dimension of life.

They also teach us that we may some day require the help of others. To be both dependent and independent is to be human. Everyone came into the world needing the help of someone else. Many of us will need help before we leave this world too. The line between "us" and "them" disappears when we accept that all of us have much in common with people who have dementia. By doing the right thing by them, we honor both them and ourselves, and we show the way for others in the future to do the right thing by us when our turn comes.

SUMMARY

When Dr. Alzheimer met Auguste Deiter a century ago, he did not have the benefit of the knowledge and insights we have today about the needs of people with dementia. As a result, Auguste unfortunately did not live the end of her life to the fullest. We must learn lessons from her sad story and apply them today to improve the lives of those in our care. We now understand that people with dementia have social and psychological needs that *can* be met. We now know they are responsive when we engage them in personal and creative ways. We now see it is possible to break through their isolation and loneliness and welcome them into a caring and encouraging community. It is now possible to thrive in the midst of dementia.

If a person-centered approach is embraced, you can no longer see people with dementia as hopeless and helpless. Negative thinking and low expectations are replaced by optimism as you see them as fully alive instead of diseased. You will become dedicated to learning the skills necessary to promote their best possible quality of life. You will gladly go about changing your attitudes and thinking to meet their needs. You will see yourself in them and treat them with the utmost respect and dignity. In doing so, your job will become a rewarding career. You will make a positive difference in the lives of others. By your example, you will teach others, like you, how to provide the best possible dementia care.

——

THINK ABOUT IT

1. Review the set of five beliefs described in this chapter. Do you agree with all of them? What are some important lessons about life and living that people with dementia have taught you?

2. Have you known someone like Auguste Deiter who seemed cut off from her own self due to dementia? What did this person say or do that affected you? Knowing what you know now, how might you have reached out to this person?

3. Can you describe three simple things that you consistently do or say that make a positive difference in the lives of your residents with dementia?

4. Think of a person you care for right now who is living with dementia—someone like Earl, Mildred or Lucinda. Based on what you have learned in this chapter, what ideas can you apply to improve this person's quality of life?

C h a p t e r

THE ARTIST OF DEMENTIA CARE

"Great art is the outward expression of an inner life in the artist."

— Edward Hopper,
American painter

MORE THAN A CAREGIVER

When you *give* care to someone, the person you care for runs the risk of becoming a passive *recipient*. This caregiver and care receiver arrangement can easily become a one-way street. You may unintentionally end up doing everything while the person you care for may do nothing. When someone's remaining abilities are overlooked or not used, helplessness and dependence may result. Personal freedom and self-esteem may be threatened. Well-being is not possible unless those you care for are actively engaged in decisions affecting them. To maximize the well-being and independence of your residents, in this chapter we introduce the highly rewarding role of artist—an artist of dementia care.

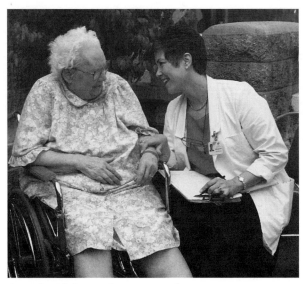

An artist of dementia care at work.

WHAT IS AN ARTIST?

An artist is a person whose work shows exceptional creative ability or skill. Maybe you are a good cook—an artist in the kitchen! Maybe you have a green thumb—an artist in the garden! Or perhaps you are engaged in other creative arts because you like to sing, act, dance, paint, sculpt, or build. Artists love their chosen field of expression and show the utmost respect for their skills and materials. Everyone holds special skills, whether they use them or are yet to develop them. Thinking as an artist of dementia care can give you a new perspective on your work with people who have dementia. When you think of your caregiving as more than a job, you become committed to learning the skills required to best serve the needs of everyone in your care. Both you and those with dementia can enjoy countless opportunities when you see yourself involved in rich and meaningful relationships. This is the art of living fully in the moment with those whom you encounter in your work.

YOU AS THE ARTIST

Unlike a well-known artist whose work of art is displayed in museums, galleries, and other public places, your work is known to only a few people—yourself and, most importantly, those entrusted into your care. They are both your critics and the ones to truly appreciate your artistry. Although your work affects a relatively small number of people at any given time, it is vitally important to each one of them. A true artist of dementia care understands the potential impact of one's artistry. The following anonymous quote sums up the vital role you may play in the lives of your residents: *"To the world you may be one person, but to one person you may be the world."*

Just as an artist's talents need to be developed to achieve a work of art, you too must develop certain personal skills and qualities to become an artist of dementia care. When you refine these skills and qualities, you are able to create overall improvement and well-being in the person with dementia. This is truly important and rewarding human work. In our view, an artist of dementia care possesses six essential skills and qualities. These include:

1. Empathy
2. Love
3. Understanding
4. Respect
5. Playfulness
6. Encouragement

These six skills are about the quality of your interactions with your residents, not the quantity or amount of time you spend with them. These skills require an attitude of *positive intention*—to do right by your residents at all times. The more you invest in this overall attitude, the more pleasure you and your residents with dementia will experience together. This positive intention will also help you to prevent many of the so-called difficult behaviors associated with dementia.

THE ESSENTIAL SKILLS OF THE ARTIST

Empathy

This skill involves seeing the world from another person's point of view. To empathize means to imagine stepping into another person's shoes and finding out what it might be like to think and feel as that other person. Inspired by Antoine De Saint-Exupéry's story, *The Little Prince,* we describe empathy in this way:

> *"What the eye sees is only a shell.*
> *What is essential is invisible to the eye.*
> *Only with the heart can we see the essential."*

In your education and training, you may have been taught to keep a professional distance from your residents. The basic aim of this idea was to avoid getting too close to them so that you would not take on their feelings of sadness, loneliness, or other negative feelings. You were supposed not to get attached to your residents to avoid "burn out." When you adopt this detached attitude, however, you view your residents from an outsider's perspective. You do not take into account how they view the world. A gap then exists between you and them.

Take, for example, Mildred, who from outward appearances has suffered significant losses and problems due to dementia. She may feel depressed by her circumstances but, if you have no emotional connection to Mildred, you may not think much about how she feels. After all, you may conclude that there is no hope left and not much to be achieved with her in any case. At best, you may try to keep her comfortable. On the other hand, if you choose to step into Mildred's shoes, you can listen with your *heart* and get to know her feelings. If you decide to have an emotional connection to her, you are likely to be motivated to do something to ease her depression. You feel responsible for trying to improve her quality of life. She becomes a special woman who has unique likes and dislikes; one who is able to love, sing, and dance; and one who can still make a difference to you and others. This shift from seeing with the eyes to seeing with your *heart* enables you to experience new possibilities.

Your work as an artist may at times seem burdensome if you cannot see something of value in people with dementia and how you can bring value to them. However, when you focus on their remaining strengths and joyful possibilities, your role as an artist can be highly rewarding. When you begin to see with your heart, you gain enormous personal satisfaction in your work. Whenever emotional barriers are removed and a meaningful relationship is established, each encounter with your residents becomes an opportunity to make a real human connection. You are bound to make a positive difference in their lives and your own life too.

To be able to step into another person's shoes you need to use your *intuition*. This refers to your lightening fast ability to process all that enters through your senses: sight, sound, smell, taste, and touch. In a split second, incoming information is tested against all that you have learned and experienced in the past. When someone asks you a question, your brain will often process two types of answers. The first one is your intuitive answer and the second is your logical answer. Intuitive responses are faster and often far more precise than logical answers. One of the most brilliant thinkers of all time, Albert Einstein, pointed out the limits of logic by remarking, "The only real valuable thing is intuition."

When you step into Mildred's shoes and see with your heart, ask yourself this question: "What strengths does she still possess?" Listen to the first answer that comes to mind; it is your intuitive response. It might be, "She is able to see the good in other people." As soon as this answer comes to mind, your logical response disputes it, "How ridiculous! Her judgment is impaired due to dementia. Of course, she can't really see the good in others." Either response may be true, depending on which perspective you choose. The first intuitive answer responds to Mildred as a person. In contrast, the second logical answer responds to Mildred in terms of her dementia symptoms. An artist of dementia care trusts the first intuitive response and acts accordingly.

Love

Upon reading the word "love" in connection with being an artist of dementia care, your initial reaction might be, "Is this a joke? Love is only for the closest and most special people in my life." Most dictionaries contain a minimum of ten definitions for different types of love. The love we speak of here is broader than the intimate bond between two people or the close ties between parents and children. Universal love refers to an affectionate dedication to others. It involves an abiding and selfless concern for the welfare of others. Sometimes this is referred to as altruism. Empathy, described above, is part of this type of love. However, there is more to love than seeing with the heart.

Love is also about compassion—the deep awareness of another person's suffering coupled with the wish to relieve it. People with dementia often lose their self-confidence and stop trying to do things

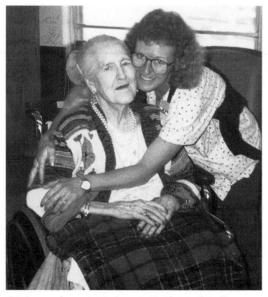

Giving and receiving love is the basis for all successful relationships.

for themselves. They may no longer see opportunities to be successful and retreat into themselves. Dr. Marshall Rosenberg described compassion as the innate desire to enrich another person's life. He posed this powerful question: "What can I do right now to make the other person's life more wonderful?" Wrestling with this question helps to focus on the needs of another person.

Love is also about forgiveness. Sometimes people with dementia may say or do things that are strange and hurtful to you. Instead of feeling upset or insulted, you can choose to forgive the person, knowing that dementia is at the root of the offending remarks. Once you allow yourself to think like this, you are free to forgive and let go.

Love is perhaps the most important human quality you can develop as an artist in dementia care. This quality needs to be an integral part of your being. Love is an act of will. It is your choice to love or not to love people with dementia.

Understanding

To truly understand people with dementia, you need to know that there is always a personal, meaningful explanation for what they do or say, no matter how strange it may seem at first. For example, Lucinda is served a sandwich, but she does not sit down at the table to eat. Instead, she stands up with the sandwich and breaks the bread into small pieces. She then throws the pieces onto the dining room floor. If you do not understand Lucinda, you are likely to interpret her behavior as inappropriate. If she repeats this behavior, you may think that she is doing this to annoy you. Now step into Lucinda's shoes and ask yourself, "What is she trying to accomplish with this behavior?" If you find this question challenging, try following Lucinda's actions step-by-step.

First, close your hand around some imaginary pieces of bread. Turn your hand around so you can see the palm of your hand with closed fingers. Now throw the imaginary bread onto the floor with several large arm movements while asking yourself, "What is Lucinda trying to accomplish?" Remember to listen to the first thought that

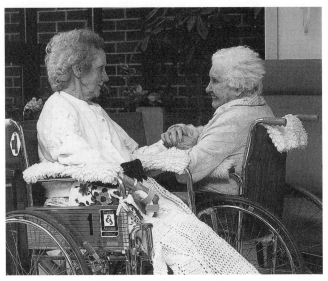

Caring for others fulfills one of our most important
emotional needs.

comes into your mind! Is it possible that she is feeding birds or
chickens? Yes, this is exactly what she appears to be doing! Why
would Lucinda feed bread to imaginary chickens on the dining room
floor?

To answer this question, you need to understand that there are
four major universal emotional needs that are frequently not fulfilled
for people with dementia. These needs are:

- To feel needed and useful
- To have an opportunity to care for someone or something
- To have one's self-esteem boosted
- To give and receive love

When these emotional needs are not met, people with dementia have
an amazing ability to recreate memories of significant people, places,
objects, or situations at a time in their past when these needs were

being met. They strive to compensate for what is now missing in their lives. In Lucinda's case, she is recreating a memory from her childhood when she had the daily job of feeding the chickens on her family's farm. When she recreated this memory, her needs to feel useful and to care for something are fulfilled. With this understanding about Lucinda's background, her behavior makes sense.

As an artist of dementia care, you find creative ways to meet Lucinda's emotional needs in this reality. You might ask her to help with the dishes, look after a pet, or prepare part of a meal or snack.

Once you seek to understand the reasons behind the seemingly strange behavior of your residents, it becomes second nature to be creative in responding to their emotional needs.

An Exercise

The following exercise will help you experience how real it is for a person with dementia who recreates an experience in one's imagination.

Using your imagination, follow these instructions, reading slowly and pausing between each step:

1. Imagine a table with a cutting board, a knife, and a lemon.
2. Take the lemon in one hand and the knife in the other hand.
3. Cut the lemon into two halves, lengthwise.
4. Take one half and cut that into two quarters.
5. Pick up one of the quarters and take a huge bite of the lemon!

What did you experience by doing this exercise? Did you see the lemon? Did you smell the lemon? Did you taste the lemon? Did you grimace? Did your mouth tingle? Whatever your responses, remember that there was no lemon! It was only your imagination recreating the memory of tasting a lemon. The mind cannot distinguish between what is real and what is imagined. For Lucinda, recreating a memory from her childhood in her imagination was as real for her as the lemon was for you.

If you look for the reason behind a behavior, you can often begin to understand it. To find the reason, check if the person with dementia is trying to fulfill one of the four emotional needs described earlier. If a need is not being met, ask yourself what you can do to help meet this need.

In order to better understand your residents, it is helpful to have information about their personal pasts. Ask family members to put together a life storybook describing major events in the person's life. Copies of old photos could highlight special memories and trigger conversations with your residents. At minimum, ask families questions about your residents' past occupations, family, and friends as well as favorite holidays, hobbies, sports, religious activities, and other interests. Be sure to ask for anecdotes that offer "snapshots" of insight into the personalities and backgrounds of your residents. Also ask about any traumas the person may have experienced, as these may resurface in old age.

In ideal circumstances, every resident's personal history should be collected and known by staff prior to admission. Family members or friends should be requested to complete a form or take part in an interview in which they are requested to share details about a loved one's past relationships, living situations, careers, hobbies, interests, religion, and so forth. Likes, dislikes, values, habits, and interesting information about the person should be documented. To the extent possible, residents should be included in the process of gathering such information. Some facilities formalize this process by asking family members and friends to put together a scrapbook that includes facts about the person's life and photos that highlight past events or special occasions. An artist of dementia care should know at least ten details about each resident. We encourage you to share this knowledge with your co-workers, volunteers, and other visitors.

It is helpful to write facts on index cards for easy access to personal information about each of your residents. These cards can be updated as needed. A card may look like the accompanying example:

Resident's Name: Mildred	**Date:** July 2007

1. Prefers to be called by her full name of Mildred.
2. Husband of 56 years, Martin.
3. Has one son and two daughters; Sally & Nancy live locally and visit often.
4. Another son, Jerry, died at age 12 in a car accident; a source of sadness.
5. Was a housewife until her kids were grown, then was a librarian.
6. Likes word games and gardening.
7. Likes coffee with milk in the morning, tea in the afternoon.
8. Loves chocolate and dislikes green vegetables.
9. Likes to wear sweaters to keep from feeling cold.
10. Private about bathing; keep a towel around her whenever possible.
11. Warm the water before Mildred steps into the shower.

Respect

To respect means to honor the essence of the person. The essence of people with dementia is not their impairments in memory, thinking, and other brain functions. Dementia does not represent the whole person. As an artist of dementia care, you can show respect in many different ways and in many different situations that honor the whole person.

People like Earl and Mildred often have trouble following conversations. You can expect a delay in their responses to questions. Respect is about giving Earl and Mildred the time they need to find the right answers. Respect is also about asking questions that they can respond to easily. You may be surprised how well Earl and

Mildred can respond once you respect their need for time and patience in conversation.

You can also show respect by cutting back on the amount of information you give at one time. For example, just imagine Mildred's confusion if you greeted her by launching into a series of statements or questions such as, "Good morning, Mildred. I am Emma. I'm here to take you to the gardening group and it starts in five minutes. Have you got your purse? Do you need a coat? By the way, your son is coming to pick you up after gardening group to take you out to lunch together with your sister." An artist of dementia care might say instead, "Good morning, Mildred. I am Emma. I'm here to invite you to the gardening group." You would then quietly assist Mildred to gather her purse and coat. Once on your way to the gardening group, you could say, "By the way, your son is coming to take you out to lunch with your sister later." It is much easier for Mildred to respond when you take the time to ask one question or give one piece of information at a time.

Respect is about the way you listen and in listening without judgment. It means taking the time to *really* hear what the other person is saying. This involves listening not just to their words but to the feelings behind the words. People with dementia are entitled to have good and bad days and to experience happiness and sadness. Although it can be hard to see or hear them "let off steam," it is important to show respect when they express negative emotions. By respectfully listening to someone's feelings, without judgment, you convey trust, acceptance, and a genuine desire to help. You do not need to offer advice. You simply need to be present and listen carefully in order to show respect.

People with dementia sometimes have unusual ways of expressing themselves or they may misinterpret the meaning of situations. It may be difficult to respect their seemingly confused ideas or misguided opinions. For example, Earl might insist that the two shirts you took from his wardrobe are both brand new and should be kept for a special occasion. If you argue that the shirts have been worn many times, he is likely to "dig his heels in" and express anger because you are challenging him. After all, these are his shirts! If you choose instead to respect Earl's reality as fact and ask him to choose another shirt, you can avoid a conflict. You might ask yourself, "Does it really matter?" If the answer is "No," then it is far better to "go along in order to get along."

To hold and show respect for people with dementia is both a skill and an attitude. It needs to be a way of life that supports every interaction you have with those you care for.

Playfulness

Playfulness is the basis of all creativity. To consistently experience fun and spontaneity is extremely important for an artist. To be an artist of dementia care, you need to be playful in order to respond effectively in a variety of challenging situations. Some of the most playful people are improvisational actors who give performances without a script or careful preparation. They usually take an idea from their audience and instantly begin to develop a humorous story. It takes self-confidence and freedom from inhibitions to be so quick on one's feet. You can learn to improvise by responding instantly and playfully to challenges posed by people like Earl, Mildred, and Lucinda. You are called upon every day to practice the art of improvisation.

Play is not just for children. Play is for everyone. It inspires our creativity, makes us laugh, and helps us learn. Playfulness builds bridges between people, cultures, and languages. It motivates us and gives us pleasure. In short, play rekindles the "spark of life." Play has these same positive effects on people with dementia too. However, there is a risk that play or playfulness can become demeaning, patronizing, or childlike for adults with dementia, but this is only when it is not combined with love and respect. When people with dementia clap, smile, laugh, and respond with joy to a playful approach, it should be interpreted positively. If they do not like a particular activity, they will let you know through verbal and non-verbal feedback. Either way, you need to respect their response.

The most successful artists of dementia care are those who use playfulness as an attitude, in close combination with unconditional love and respect for people with dementia. They use spontaneity, joy, humor, and fun. They communicate positive regard for others. They are comfortable with their own inner child. They are not inhibited by what others think about them or their approach. They are comfortable initiating a dance with Earl because he loves to waltz. They enjoy using pictures to create stories with Mildred because she has a vivid imagination. They happily massage Lucinda's body because it's the only time she smiles with pleasure. Louise Hay described the benefits of play for both parties when she wrote, "The child in me knows how to play and love and wonder . . . it opens the door to my heart, and my life is enriched."

Encouragement

Dementia threatens the self-esteem and identity of your residents due to their increasing impairments and dependence on others. They may feel worthless or burdensome. Your role is to offer them encouragement so they can overcome their loss of self-esteem. To encourage someone means to inspire with confidence or to give hope and courage.

If you think of self-esteem as a bank account, your residents struggle to keep a positive balance. If a deposit is made, the balance goes up, but if there is a withdrawal, the balance comes down. Whenever you or I succeed at something—no matter how small—and that

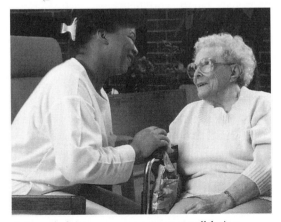

Acknowledging success promotes well-being.

success is acknowledged in a genuine way, our self-esteem account increases. However, the self-esteem account can be drawn down by negative experiences. If you make a suggestion of how to solve a problem only to have your effort squashed by others, your self-esteem may diminish. After awhile, your self-esteem account may drop so low that you don't wish to take a risk again. This is also true for people with dementia. Depression and social isolation may become a way of life. They may retreat into a private world where they feel safe and free of failure. However, you can prevent this from happening by boosting their self-esteem. An artist of dementia care reaches out and helps them feel worthwhile again by encouraging them to use their remaining strengths and abilities.

To offer encouragement, it is helpful to shift your focus from the many things that your residents can no longer do well (such as remembering recent events, using fluent language, and dressing independently) to the many things that they are still able to do successfully. Begin by thinking of one person with dementia whom you know well. Can this person smile, laugh, sing, clap, drink, or say hello? What else can this person do? Write down a list of at least ten different things so you can encourage the use of these remaining abilities or strengths.

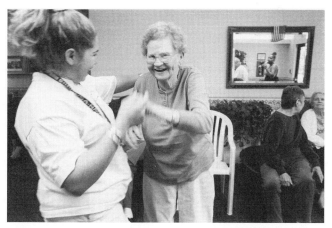

Dancing may be just one of many remaining abilities.
© Cathy Stein Greenblat

To encourage your residents, an artist of dementia care takes active steps to empower and enable them to achieve their highest potential. You give them confidence and ensure that they can keep doing what they can for as long as possible. You can do this by becoming aware of the little things that the person with dementia can still do for oneself. You ensure success by assisting as needed. You encourage the use of abilities and compensate for disabilities of residents like Earl, Mildred, and Lucinda.

Earl, who is in the early stages of dementia, may still have the initiative to ask if there is anything he can do to help. It is important to offer him a real job; one that is meaningful to him. On the other hand, Earl may lack initiative yet readily respond to your request for help with a specific task. If his self-esteem is low from repeated instances of past failure, he may need encouragement to try again. You might ask him if he could give you a hand with something that is meaningful to him, such as sorting through the mail (you can have a special pile of mail ready for Earl), or sweeping the floor. Remember to sincerely thank him for his help. His self-esteem account will increase as a result of your encouragement.

Mildred, who is in the middle stages of dementia, may need to be talked through each step of a task in more detail than Earl. She may lack confidence that she can do anything right and may easily give up on the task. She needs more encouragement than someone like Earl. You might invite her to fold napkins, one at a time, rather than expect her to complete the entire job on her own. As she finishes one task, you sincerely thank her for helping and encourage her to continue until finished. Her self-esteem will be boosted.

Lucinda, who is in the late stage, still enjoys singing, although she rarely sings on her own. Perhaps she cannot recall the words to start a song. You could take the lead and sing her favorite song while encouraging her to join you. You can then thank her for brightening your day with her song. You can repeat this ritual several times a day and further validate Lucinda's identity as a singer. Your encouragement may inspire her to feel good about herself.

In any of the above scenarios, you could argue that there is not enough time or enough staff for this kind of personal attention. After all, you are a busy person. You may be in a hurry with all sorts of tasks and think that such attention will probably slow you down. But what is the point of completing these tasks if your residents do not benefit and experience self-esteem? Instead of feeling cared for, they may feel diminished by the fact that you are taking away their power to do things for themselves. Therefore, providing encouragement to your residents is one of your most important roles as an artist of dementia care. It is perhaps the best way to boost their self-esteem and help them maintain their personal identity.

SUMMARY

This chapter focused on the essential qualities and skills needed in order to become an excellent artist of dementia care. You may already hold all of these qualities and skills. However, the savvy artist knows that there is always room for improvement and much more to learn. One does not perfect the art of dementia care in a week, a month, or a year. It takes constant practice and refinement to make it a part of yourself and to apply this art on a daily basis. The American educator Marva Collins once said, "Excellence is not an act but a habit. The things you do the most are the things you will do the best." We hope that the skills of the artist of dementia care will become so ingrained in your life that they will become natural habits, not a set of techniques. This will enrich not only the lives of those in your care, but also your own.

To further your thinking about the person-centered approach as the basis for being an artist of dementia care, we turn now to how this positive approach differs to the medical approach that dominates long-term care today.

THINK ABOUT IT

1. What does logical thinking tell you about the limits and losses of those people in your care?
2. What does your intuition tell you about their remaining strengths and abilities?
3. How did you feel when someone showed you empathy during a particularly difficult time in your life?
4. Think of one resident who is withdrawn, sad, or irritable. What can you do right now to improve this person's life?
5. Recall an incident in which a resident was verbally or physically aggressive toward you. How did you forgive this person? If you have not yet forgiven this person, can you let go of your resentment?
6. Are your residents given daily opportunities to help with their own care, the care of others, or other productive tasks? And then, are they sincerely thanked for their contributions?

SHIFTING THOUGHTS, WORDS, AND ACTIONS

"Kindness in thinking creates profoundness. Kindness in words creates confidence. Kindness in giving creates love."
— Lao Tzu,
Chinese philosopher

THE PERSON-CENTERED APPROACH

The person-centered approach involves helping people who have dementia to improve or maximize their well-being. This approach represents a radical shift from the traditional approach that is common in residential care facilities. Dementia has long been viewed mainly as a medical problem—an irreversible, progressive, and hopeless disorder of the brain. In the medical approach, little can be done for the unfortunate "patients" since there is no cure and few drugs for treating their symptoms. In the medical approach, difficult behaviors expressed by people with dementia, such as agitation, are seen as inevitable symptoms due to brain damage. This approach is pessimistic in its outlook and ignores the importance of good care on the well-being of people with dementia. In contrast, a person-centered approach is optimistic and dementia care is seen as important and uplifting work.

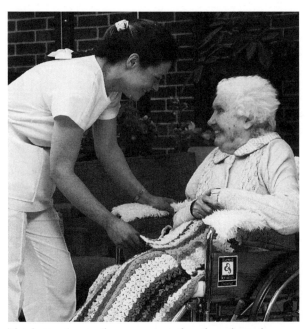

Total attention to the person—rather than the task—
creates well-being.

A person-centered approach views dementia mainly in terms of
its psychological and social effects on the person who has a disability. The person-centered approach assumes that much can be done
to help people with dementia to enjoy their lives in spite of problems
with memory, thinking, language, and so forth. Their "difficult
behaviors" are not seen as inevitable symptoms of their illness, but
as signs of personal distress or other unmet needs. The manner in
which people with dementia are cared for in their social environment
makes all the difference. This approach requires that those who support people with dementia must take responsibility for ensuring their
well-being. Once you make this shift in thinking from the medical
approach to a person-centered approach, you begin to change your
outlook as well your language and actions so that people with
dementia can better cope with their limitations.

WHAT IS YOUR PERSPECTIVE?

The medical approach emphasizes the limits to your efforts, while the person-centered approach recognizes that you have an important role to play in contributing to the well-being of your residents. Although an artist of dementia care will choose to focus on the needs of each person, it is easy to get caught up in the predominant way of thinking that focuses on dementia as a medical condition. Which approach you adopt is strongly determined by where you focus your attention. Your focus will shape your ideas, feelings, words, and actions. The following example illustrates this point.

Imagine three passengers on a bus. One is a man riding this bus for the first time. He has to get off at the stop where there is a McDonald's™ restaurant on one corner and a gas station on the other. He is busy focusing his attention on looking out and waiting for these places to appear. The second passenger is an older lady who loves to ride the bus purely for the enjoyment of looking out the window at people's gardens. The third passenger is a young woman who enjoys making up stories about fellow passengers—why they are on the bus; where they are going; and what is happening in their lives.

Imagine that these three passengers board the bus at the same time and get off at the same stop where the McDonald's™ restaurant is located. Although the three passengers completed the same trip, each will have had a different experience. Each passenger held a different focus during the trip. If we asked the young woman who made up stories or the man who was on the bus for the first time if they could tell us about the gardens they passed, they would have no idea. What each person focused on determined his or her own unique experience.

If you focus on dementia as an irreversible and progressive disorder, you will think only about someone's deterioration of abilities. You may have been led to believe that dementia is a hopeless condition. You may think to yourself, "Dementia drags the person downhill. No matter what I do or how much I try, people with dementia will get worse." Or you may be a bit more optimistic and think, "If I truly support people with dementia, I may help maintain their current level of ability." In either case, you have low expectations of your residents. You will also have low expectations of your own ability to do much for them, except for providing physical care.

On the other hand, if you focus on dementia as a breakdown of certain parts of the brain, you are more likely to see dementia in a different way. You do not become upset over things your residents say or do because you know there is an underlying reason. You are in touch with their emotional needs and respond compassionately. It is possible for you to improve their ability to cope with the problems they are experiencing. You take responsibility for creating an atmosphere that enables your residents to thrive every day. You know there is hope for making a positive difference in their lives. You can make this happen through your ideas, feelings, words, and actions.

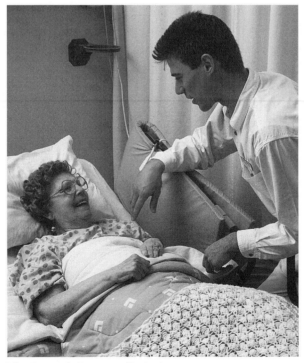

Think possibilities, not limitations.

Rehabilitation specialists are accustomed to enacting positive change among persons who have physical disabilities. First, they work on minimizing the disabling condition to ensure the highest level of the individual's functioning. Second, they strengthen the person's other abilities to compensate for any limits. Rehabilitation may not restore a person's memory, thinking, and other brain functions. However, there is much that can be done to minimize and compensate for limits and enhance remaining skills or abilities. Too often dementia is associated with doom and gloom. Thinking in terms of a person with disability means that you focus on the individual's possibilities instead of their limitations or impairments.

The feelings, thoughts, and words you use in your inner dialogue or when speaking to others have a profound effect on your actions and the results you are able to achieve. Imagine looking at a bottle with half of its contents—is it half full or half empty? If you think of the bottle as half full, then you are likely to feel better about how much remains rather than focusing on what is missing. In short, what you think will affect how you feel. How you feel will affect how you act. And how you act will affect how another person responds.

Positive Thoughts → Positive Feelings → Positive Actions → Positive Reactions

Your thoughts, feelings, and actions are likely to determine the reactions of others. People with dementia will often reflect back your attitudes and the atmosphere you create. This is about cause and effect. Everything you do or say will have a corresponding effect. An artist of dementia care takes responsibility for the results they create—for the consequences of their actions.

CREATING A POSITIVE CULTURE

The feelings, thoughts, language, and behaviors that are shared in common by staff in residential care facilities are sometimes referred to as the "culture of care." This includes the routines and practices that are passed on from generation to generation of new staff. The culture that exists today, for the most part, is not favorable toward people with dementia. Unfortunately, the combination of negative thoughts, words, and behavior among staff members can result in breeding loneliness, helplessness, and boredom among residents. Staff members like you do not intend to create these conditions, but the culture of care is so strong that it is sometimes difficult to imagine anything else. An artist of dementia care is committed to changing this culture of care. You make it your personal business through ideas, words, and actions to ensure that the person with dementia comes first.

Labels are often used as a shorthand method of describing people with dementia. However, labels are usually demeaning and create a division between "them" and "us." Even simple words like "patient" or "resident" suggest that someone is to be treated as a set of symptoms or care needs. These labels keep us from engaging with people as individuals in need of empathy, love, and respect. Many other labels are even more dehumanizing, such as Wanderers, Feeders, Sundowners, and Screamers. These words do not describe individual human beings but rather how certain behaviors or needs are inconvenient or disruptive to care providers. If someone described you with such words, you would probably feel less than human. Yet powerful labels are often used today to define people with dementia. In a person-centered approach, someone should never be described in terms of a behavior or a need. An artist of dementia care avoids using labels and instead looks for ways to describe an individual and sees certain behaviors as expressions of unmet needs.

The label Wanderer suggests that the person walks around aimlessly, with no apparent purpose. Some people believe that wandering is a symptom of dementia. However, wandering can be seen in another light. Perhaps it is a search for someone or something from their past or an escape from a noisy or confusing environment. Perhaps it is a means to burn off energy or a way to fight boredom. If you place the term "wandering" in a positive light as simply "strolling," you are forced to consider that this behavior may be

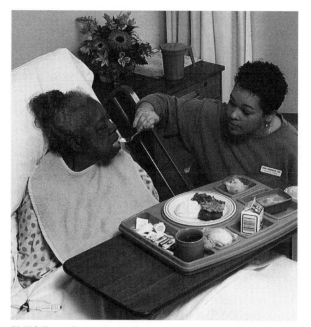

Skillfully assisting Lucinda to eat encourages her participation.

normal under the circumstances. However, if you believe there is discomfort or distress associated with a person's persistent need to walk, it is up to you to discover what is needed to relieve any discomfort or distress and to take appropriate action.

Likewise, the label Feeder is dehumanizing and should be changed to descriptive language. For example, instead of asking, "Who is doing the Feeders today?" the artist of dementia care would say, "Who is assisting Lucinda with her lunch today?" People with dementia do not like being dependent upon others for assistance with eating, and being referred to as Feeders reinforces the idea that they are considered burdensome. Instead of a label, a description is more humane. These are individuals who happen to need partial or full assistance with their meals. A shift in language encourages active participation and accepts that those who need your help will be supported in a caring and compassionate manner.

The label Sundowners conjures up images of restless, agitated people who want to go home during the late afternoon or early evening. But there may be better explanations than thinking of "sundowning" as just another symptom of dementia. At day's end, all creatures on earth return home: birds to their nests, rabbits to their warrens, and bees to their hives. Humans also return home at the end of the day. It is a daily ritual. If people with dementia do not feel like they are at home in their care facility, they will naturally look for home at the end of the day. Distress is a normal reaction to feeling lost and out of place. The current environment may not feel familiar, so home must be found elsewhere. It is up to the artist of dementia care to correctly interpret such distress and respond by offering residents a sense of comfort, safety, and home.

Perhaps most troubled and troubling are the people sometimes labeled the Screamers. As soon as you think about them, you imagine loud, anguished voices that penetrate your bones and make you cringe. This type of behavior is often considered another difficult symptom of dementia. But why does someone scream? Is there an explanation or reason? There may be untreated pain due to an aching joint, a decayed tooth, a fractured bone, or infected skin. There are many possibilities that need to be explored. Because your residents may not have the ability to form words to express discomfort, screaming may be the only way to communicate pain. People who scream are better described as individuals who are experiencing some form of physical or emotional need. By looking for potential causes of this behavior, you can take responsibility and do something about meeting the unmet need.

COMMUNICATION REQUIRES SKILLS

Communication is the exchange of information, ideas, and emotions. It is how thoughts, wishes, and feelings are conveyed to others. In order for communication to occur, a message must be sent and received. This involves speaking clearly and listening closely. You need to not only hear a message, but to understand it, too. Otherwise, communication does not take place.

People with dementia experience many communication challenges. The inability to understand or to be understood is extremely frustrating and often triggers anger, depression, and other troubled emotions. Communication breakdown is a major influence on the types of challenging behaviors we will address in the next chapter. As an artist in dementia care, you can understand the challenges in speaking and listening that face people with dementia. You know that they can still express themselves and you learn to interpret their fractured speech and non-verbal cues. You take the time to learn each person's communication sytle. You find creative ways to connect with them.

In the later stages, their words and sentences may become jumbled or they may stop talking altogether. It would be easy to think: "These people don't know how to communicate. They cannot talk or listen." If you accept this belief as fact, you are off the hook—you do not have to initiate conversation or take responsibility for enabling them to understand. Another way of looking at the situation is to consider that people with dementia are still capable of communicating yet not in customary ways. They rely less on words and more on non-verbal ways to express themselves—body language, sounds, and actions. Such an explanation encourages you to find ways to communicate in terms they understand. An artist of dementia care knows how to listen and respond to different forms of communication. Some people liken it to learning a new language.

Professor Albert Mehrabian, known for his pioneering work in the field of human communication, discovered that the meaning of our words is mainly communicated non-verbally. He found that only 7 percent of communication comes through words, 38 percent is through voice and the way words are spoken, and 55 percent is through body language, including facial expression and eye contact. Thus, 93 percent of communication does not rely upon spoken words. Non-verbal communication skills are far more effective than verbal skills! People with dementia slowly lose the ability to use and interpret words, but they still know how to communicate non-verbally. When their ability to speak and understand language falters, the tone of your voice and your facial expressions take on increasing importance.

LISTENING SKILLS

The following five ideas will help improve your listening skills when a resident is communicating with you.

Make Contact

Use your body language to show the person you are truly listening. Bend or kneel down so you are at the same eye level. Look directly into the person's eyes in a warm and welcoming way. Establish a physical connection to let the person know that you are offering your full attention.

Read Body Language

Keeping in mind that non-verbal communication can be more telling than words, focus on the resident's body language: facial expressions, gestures, posture, and touch. If you study a person's body language

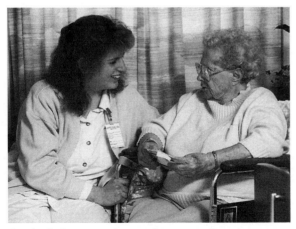

Our body language shows when we are listening to someone.

carefully, you will pick up on a great deal of information about what an individual may be thinking or feeling. At first, the clues may be subtle but as you improve your observational skills you will become well versed in "reading" another person's body language.

Make a Guess

Now you need to guess what the person is attempting to communicate. Body language and key words may offer you some clues. Based on your personal knowledge of each resident, you may have a good idea of what is a central theme or concern. Acknowledge what it is you think that the person is attempting to communicate through words, sounds, or gestures.

Check Your Guess

Ensure that what you have guessed is also true for the person with dementia. Ask questions that will require only a "yes" or "no" answer; they are much easier to respond to than open-ended questions. Here are some examples:

- "Earl, when you say you want to go home . . . is it that you are feeling lonely right now?"
- "Mildred, when you say you are looking for your mother . . . is it that you are looking for someone to make you comfortable?"
- "Lucinda, when you tap your fingers hard on the table . . . is it that you are feeling angry?"

The worst thing that can happen is that your guess is incorrect. Simply try again.

Interpret Symbolic Actions

When people with dementia communicate in nonverbal ways rather than in words, they sometimes behave in unusual ways. These actions may represent a feeling or concern. A resident may be "saying" something personally important through one's behavior. For example, Mildred clutches onto her purse at all times. When you ask her if you may place the purse on a table, she responds in an angry tone. The purse may have come to represent Mildred's identity or may give her a sense of security. It is important to respect her need to hold on to that purse!

SPEAKING SKILLS

The following six ideas will help when you are speaking with a resident. Remember: it is always the responsibility of the communicator to ensure that the message gets through to the other person.

Make Contact

Establishing contact is the key to starting any conversation. Connect with your eyes and address the person by name in a clear voice. Use the resident's preferred name; for example, George or Mr. Smith. Be genuine. Greet the resident with a smile and a calm, cheerful voice. Identify yourself—the resident may not remember you. Make sure that you can be heard! Is a hearing aid in place? Is the environment free of noisy distractions? Now wait for the person with dementia to respond before any further communication takes place.

Ask the Right Question

Have you ever organized an outing, a party or a sing-along for people with dementia? When asked to attend, they often refuse to come to this pleasant event. Sometimes the refusal is said politely, as in, "No, thank you. I am busy waiting for my son to come." Other times, it may be a sharp, "No! Leave me alone." The negative reply is often due to the manner in which the question is asked. All that is heard by someone with dementia may be, "Would you like to . . . ?" The question is interpreted as a request to do something new or unfamiliar. Rather than take a chance on something unclear or strange, it is reasonable to decline and stay in one's comfort zone. It is much safer to turn down your offer, no matter how much you think it may be beneficial.

You can turn this situation around with something that usually works—an invitation. Instead of asking, "Would you like . . ?" you say, "Earl, I have come to invite you to an outing. I would like you to be my guest." Think about the difference between being asked versus being invited. An invitation implies that you are special and that you are needed. It implies a relationship and an activity that is important to you. An invitation is associated with good feelings so that a positive response is likely. Keep in mind that it is not enough to get the wording right—you need to truly mean what you say when you extend an invitation.

Choose Positive Words

To make sure that you remain positive and supportive at all times, think consciously about the quality of the words you use in addressing your residents. Instead of asking them questions that test their memory, you can set a good tone with each new encounter. Never, ever say, "Do you remember me?" Or even worse, "Don't you remember me?" Instead, begin with a proper introduction by saying, "Good morning, Lucinda. I am (your name)." You then state your purpose such as, "I am here to assist you today." You may continue on a cheerful note by saying, "I am so glad to see you," instead of asking "How are you?"

A positive tone can also be set when you need to engage your residents in a task. Never say, "I have come to clean you up or to give you a shower." Instead, establish that you are there to offer support by announcing, "I have come to see if there is anything you need." You may then offer a choice by asking questions such as, "While I am here, what if I give you a hand making your bed? While I am here, can I give you a hand to get into the shower? While I am here, can I give you a hand brushing your dentures?" The basic idea is to provide residents with choices and opportunities for involvement on their own terms. If they see themselves as objects of your help, instead of active participants in their own care, they are less likely to participate in a task or activity.

Use Simple Words and a Slow Pace

People with dementia process information more slowly than they did in the past. Be sure not to outpace them and use words they can understand. Concrete words that you can picture are best instead of abstract words that can be difficult to comprehend. Above all, be brief. If you go on and on, they will lose track of what you are saying. You may have to break a conversation or instructions into steps. Introduce ideas or instructions one thing at a time. Allow plenty of time for a response. If you get a dazed or uncertain look in response, it is a sign that what you have said has not been understood. For example, instead of asking, "Would you like something to eat?" narrow down the question with two choices: "May I get you a cup of tea or coffee?" Wait patiently for a response. It is in the pause—in the silence—that communication happens.

Use Different Sensory Cues

The five human senses involve seeing, hearing, touching, tasting, and smelling. If at all possible, use different senses to communicate. Use gestures and visual prompts to reinforce what you are saying with your words. For example, a towel and a washcloth can help introduce that it is time to take a shower.

Physical contact can be reassuring and help get a message across. If the person does not mind, gently touch a hand or arm to literally make a connection. Most people with dementia in the middle and later stages, when language skills diminish, seem to enjoy a hug. So that your hug is really felt, make sure it lasts for at least 7 seconds. Then both the giver and the receiver of the hug will know that it is really genuine. If someone appears reluctant to receive a hug, you might ask, "I really need a hug—could I have a hug?" In asking for a hug, you remind the person with dementia that he or she is needed, able to care for someone, and has an opportunity to give as well as receive affection. Whenever you use touch to communicate, be aware of the signs when someone enjoys touch and when it is not enjoyed. Signs of enjoyment include relaxed facial muscles and shoulders and deep or slowed breathing. Signs of discomfort include muscle tension and shallow or anxious breathing. When used appropriately, touch can speak volumes about your care and concern for others. Remember that it is not what you do, but the way that you do it that counts.

Use Reminiscence

A person with dementia typically loses short-term memory but retains memories from the distant past until the late stages of dementia. Although your residents may not remember what they had for breakfast, they may well remember their lives as children or young adults. Reminiscence or recalling past experiences in conversation may help to maintain or improve their verbal abilities. Although you may grow tired of hearing their old stories being repeated, for them, it may be like they are telling the story for the very first time. Pleasurable memories can bring the past to life again and create much joy in the present.

Reminiscence is a way of tapping into well-preserved memories from long ago. Apart from encouraging residents to talk about the past, you can use different senses to evoke memories. The sense of sight can be used to examine and talk about old pictures and photographs. The sense of hearing can be used to listen and respond to music from the past. The sense of touch can be used to handle memorabilia, such as an antique, a baby doll, or an old tool. The sense of smell can be used to evoke memories with different aromas and oils. The sense of taste can also bring treasured memories into the present, such as home-baked chocolate chip cookies. The five senses can be used to tap into the past and bring them into the here and now.

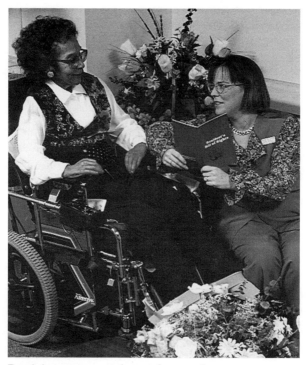

Reminiscence can evoke good memories.

When you are sitting with Mildred looking at old photos, objects, or treasures, never ask factual questions such as, "Where was this photo taken? What is this called? Who took this photo?" All such questions require precise answers and may easily confuse Mildred. Instead, here are some questions you can ask that encourage Mildred to have an enjoyable conversation.

- What do you see in this picture?
- What does this picture say to you?
- How do you feel when you look at this picture?
- What do you think about this picture?

These are powerful questions because they can yield many different responses. No matter what Mildred answers to any of them—her answers are always going to be right! Such questions guarantee that she will have a successful interaction.

SUMMARY

From your experience, you understand that people with dementia do not think or behave in "normal" ways. In response, you have learned to adjust your own thoughts, feelings, and behaviors to adjust to their needs. You no longer expect them, for example, to remember your name and instead tell them about yourself. You take responsibility for enabling them to use their remaining skills. By making these adjustments, you can save yourself and your residents much frustration.

In this chapter, you have been challenged to create opportunities for your residents to experience enjoyment. As you once shifted your thoughts, feelings, and actions to minimize the frustration of your residents, you can grow even further by thinking, feeling, and acting in more positive ways. An artist of dementia care knows how to set off a chain reaction of pleasurable moments for residents with dementia. This begins by first developing an optimistic outlook that is then communicated in words and actions to others. If you believe that nothing can be done for people with dementia, they will experience your pessimism. If you believe that much can be done to maintain or enhance their well-being, they will experience your optimism through your words, feelings, and actions.

THINK ABOUT IT

1. When other people find out that you care for people with dementia and state that this must be depressing work, how do you respond? Do you basically agree with them or do you challenge them to think differently about your supportive role and responsibilities?

2. How does your faith, your family, or your past experiences influence your outlook toward dementia and people with dementia?
3. What are your favorite ways for listening or speaking to people with dementia? What are some additional ways to expand your communication skills?

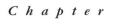

HOW TO TURN AROUND CHALLENGING BEHAVIORS

"Understanding human needs is half the job of meeting them."
—Adlai Stevenson,
American statesman

Sometimes people with dementia say or do things that are undesirable and unpleasant for themselves, you, other staff members, other residents, families, or other visitors. Some examples of these challenging behaviors include abusive or insulting language, aggression, physical resistance to care, refusal to cooperate, and verbal outbursts. Coping with such behaviors may be the most demanding part of your work. An artist of dementia care steps into the shoes of the person with dementia to find out why these behaviors occur. This person-centered approach enables you to see difficult behaviors as:

1. **Reactions.** Instead of jumping to the conclusion that the person you care for is being difficult on purpose, think of these behaviors as a reaction to something that isn't right for that individual. From his or her point of view, these behaviors are reasonable responses to pain, fear, or other unwelcome feelings.

2. **Expressions of Unmet Needs.** Underlying all difficult behaviors is a physical, social, spiritual, or emotional need that is not being met. People with dementia often do not have the means to express their needs in customary ways. Thus, their behaviors are attempts to communicate unmet needs.

YOU CAN HELP

If you think of difficult behaviors strictly as symptoms of dementia, then they are out of your control—you have no responsibility for addressing the underlying reason. However, if you think of difficult behaviors as reactions and expressions of needs, then they become your personal business. This is an important distinction. An artist of dementia care knows that people with dementia have little or no control over their challenging behaviors. If they could reason, remember, and talk about what was bothering them instead of expressing themselves in unpleasant ways, they would choose to do so. Whatever they say or do now has become a new type of "normal" for them. As a result, you accept people with dementia the way they are—good or bad, pleasant or unpleasant, easy or challenging.

With an accepting attitude, you do your best to understand their thoughts, feelings, and actions. This attitude enables you to look for the causes or triggers of their challenging behaviors and to develop creative solutions. You do not have to do this alone. You can share your ideas with your supervisor or other staff members so that all of you work together to find the best approach. As your detective skills grow, you may become so adept at interpreting challenging behaviors that you can actually begin to prevent them from happening in the first place.

Instead of seeing challenging behaviors as problems, an artist of dementia care sees them as opportunities for meeting the unmet needs of people with dementia. At any given moment, you have the power to see either problems or opportunities. Again, it all depends

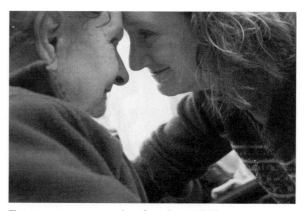

Eye to eye contact makes for a beautiful human connection. © Cathy Stein Greenblat

upon your attitude or perspective. To illustrate this shift in thinking, consider the work of Michelangelo (1475–1564) who was one of the world's greatest, multi-talented artists: a musician, poet, architect, painter, and sculptor. As a sculptor, his preferred material was white marble. When embarking on his angel, David, Michelangelo did not focus on the block of white marble in front of him. Instead, he saw through the marble to an angel trapped inside. He chiseled away to free the angel and his masterpiece was born.

This analogy represents the essence—the core of being a true artist of dementia care. The artist's eye does not stop at face value. The artist's eye sees deeper to the possibilities within each person. In cases of difficult behavior, the artist of dementia care looks beyond the behavior to the trapped angel and recognizes that it represents an unmet need.

KNOW YOURSELF

There is no substitute for knowing your residents in order to understand what may trigger their challenging behaviors. Their unique preferences, coping styles, moods, and personal histories should be familiar to you. Each person's abilities and limitations should be well understood. This personal information is invaluable for detecting what might be wrong and how you can help. Apart from familiarity and knowledge about each of your residents, the most important tool you possess for turning around difficult behaviors is yourself.

Self-awareness is critical for the artist of dementia care. Challenging behaviors are opportunities to hold up a mirror and learn something about yourself. These situations often reveal how you feel about yourself, your relationships, your beliefs, your sense of humor, your sensitivity, and your self-confidence. These personal thoughts and feelings influence how you interpret challenging situations and shape your responses. If you do not feel good about yourself or your residents, you are likely to respond with mistrust or dislike. If you feel good about yourself and those in your care, you are likely to respond with understanding and compassion. Your attitude or perspective, and not your residents' behavior, is the key.

Imagine for a moment that you are walking down a wide corridor at your care facility. Walking toward you is the one person who gives you the shivers—your most difficult resident—the one you would really like to avoid. As you pass each other, this other person brushes against you. A tremor of discomfort runs through your body. You think to yourself: That was deliberate and unacceptable behavior.

Now imagine that you are again walking down the same wide corridor but, this time, it is a different person coming toward you. Imagine a movie star who is extremely attractive. You cannot avoid gazing at this person. As you pass each other, this good-looking person brushes against you. What runs through your mind this time? Could it be that your response to this second person is different from your response to the first person? Most likely, the answer is yes. In fact, you may even be thrilled by this brief encounter.

This example shows that it is not the behavior itself that is difficult. It is your interpretation of the behavior that makes all the difference. If you are inclined to see a problem, you will see it. If you are inclined to see an opportunity, you will see it. The choice is yours to make.

How you feel about another person will affect your interpretation of that person's behavior too. Think about the people you care for. It is likely that there are some who can get away with certain behaviors that others cannot. When you look inward, what accounts for the difference? Why can one person say or do something that does not bother you when another person who says or does the same thing really irritates you? Behavior is not a problem or difficult or challenging until you interpret it as such.

When a challenging behavior does not irritate you but is agitating other residents and staff members, you are the one who can help turn the situation around for them. Because you are not consumed by negative emotion, you can devote your energy to finding out the source of the challenging behavior and work toward a solution. Instead of reacting in a defensive manner, like others, you look for the meaning behind the challenging behavior and try to address the unmet need that is being expressed in an unpleasant way. As an artist of dementia care, you are always looking through the seemingly inappropriate or strange behaviors to discover the needs that have not been met.

BEHAVIORS ARE REACTIONS

An artist of dementia care also understands that challenging behaviors can be reactions to something that is distressing. Therefore, you do not take challenging behaviors personally. You can refrain from responding to someone's anger with anger of your own. You can keep your cool because you know that something has triggered the challenging behavior. Your task is to find out what the trigger is and, if at all possible, eliminate the root cause.

Consider the following problem and how you might handle it. Your neighbor is throwing a party. Rock music is blaring, guests are loud, and now it is well past midnight. You are tired and cannot sleep. What would you do? You have many options, such as asking the neighbor to keep the noise down, putting in some earplugs, or complaining to the police. If one way fails, you may try another.

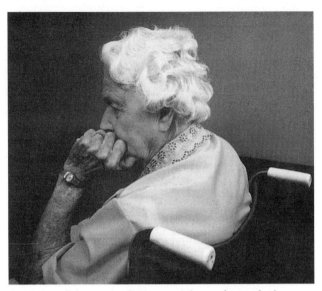

An artist of dementia eliminates sights and sounds that trigger confusion, anxiety, or fear.

In a similar situation, step into the shoes of one of your residents with dementia. You have been taken to a crowded room for a concert in the care facility. There are many confusing sights and sounds. Music is playing loudly and you dislike the type of music being played. You are tired and want to rest. You cannot tell anyone that you don't want to be there and you cannot walk out. You do not know how to get back to your room. What are your options? What means do you have to express how you are feeling? Without your usual inhibitions, how might you act in response? Is there a chance you might call out loudly, scream or swear? Perhaps even lash out? How might others respond to you?

There is always a meaningful reason behind the behavior of someone with dementia that is troubling to you or others. Your role is to find out the triggering cause and to develop a constructive solution. You can choose to react with your own negative feelings or respond compassionately. You can choose to become defensive or to be a problem solver.

Any number of things may trigger challenging behaviors. Sometimes your verbal messages are confusing to someone like Earl and he may become angry with you. Instead of becoming defensive or getting angry with him, ask yourself some questions that may explain your role in Earl's negative response:

- Was my body language warm and friendly?
- Did I make eye contact before I began to speak?
- Was I being heard?
- Did I pause after asking each question?
- Was the environment too noisy?
- Did I speak slowly and clearly?
- Did I use simple words?
- Did I ask yes/no questions?
- Did I talk respectfully?

What might I have done to block communication and trigger a negative response? Did my communication skills fall short in this situation? Can changing my behavior turn around the resident's behavior? Check yourself with this sort of self-examination. It's like holding up a mirror. If you are responsible for a breakdown in communication, you can take corrective action and minimize your resident's distress. You will also have learned how to prevent such behavior in the future.

BEHAVIORS ARE ATTEMPTS TO COMMUNICATE NEEDS

All behaviors, even the most challenging types, need to be understood as attempts to communicate by people with dementia. Distressing behaviors may be their way of saying, verbally or non-verbally, that an important need is not being met. Behind everything a person with dementia may say or do—no matter how strange it appears to you—there is always a reason that is meaningful to that individual. Rather than thinking that someone with dementia is "acting out" through angry remarks or hostile acts, you know that such behaviors are expressions of unmet needs. Sometimes the unmet need is not evident, as in the case of someone who screams for no apparent reason. Upon closer inspection, the person may be experiencing a great deal of pain. Without the ability to describe one's pain, the need for pain relief is expressed through screaming.

Like a good detective, you must discover the unmet need that triggered the behavior and then find a way to meet that need. First, stop what you are doing to consider possible explanations. Then look around and listen—what may be contributing to the behavior? There could be several triggers:

- a physical reason
- an emotional reason
- a troubling element in the environment
- a complex task or activity

A person with dementia may no longer know how to take care of one's health and well-being. Something as simple as knowing how to find and drink a glass of water may become a complex challenge. Initiating a pleasant activity to avoid boredom may seem impossible. As a result, others like you must identify and meet the physical and emotional needs of people with dementia. If their basic needs for physical and emotional comfort are not met, challenging behaviors are likely to arise.

PHYSICAL REASONS

The most common physical problem is pain. Crying out for help and screaming are signs that pain due to a medical condition may be the underlying issue. It may be difficult to pinpoint the exact cause of pain at times. A number of root causes are possible: a urinary tract infection, constipation, an adverse side effect to medication, an aching joint, a broken bone or some other medical problem. There may simply be a need to use the bathroom. If you think that pain is an issue, report your observation to someone who is in a position to investigate it further. Assessment may reveal that treatment is necessary with physical therapy, massage, medication, healing touch, or another pain relieving solution. In the end, relief is all that matters to someone with dementia. It is too bad that sometimes screaming may be the only way to get the medical attention or care that is required.

Fatigue is also a common problem that can trigger agitation and other challenging behavior. People with dementia appear to tire

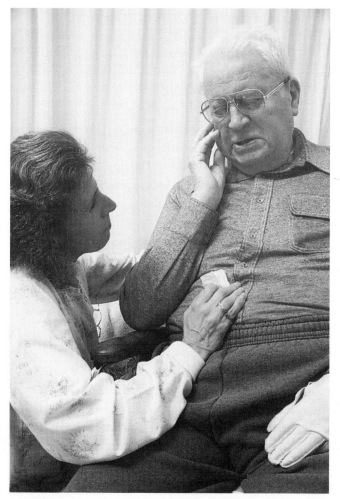

An artist of dementia care seeks to discover the need behind a behavior.

easily after a seemingly light level of physical activity. Many have trouble sleeping at night, causing daytime drowsiness. Treating sleep problems and allowing time for plenty of rest can alleviate fatigue. Hunger and thirst also cannot be overlooked. Offering snacks and water or other nutritious food and drink may resolve these problems. Vision and hearing problems can also trigger challenging behaviors. Imagine the confusion caused by not being able to see or hear what is going on around you. Replacing a hearing aid battery is sometimes the only thing necessary to ease someone's agitation!

EMOTIONAL REASONS

Unmet emotional needs can be just as important as unmet physical needs in triggering challenging behaviors. When any of the four universal emotional needs described in Chapter 2 are not met, it will often result in difficult behavior. To avoid or minimize the effects of such unmet needs, ask yourself the following questions:

1. How can I enable this person to feel needed and useful?
2. How can I enable this person to care for someone or something?
3. How can I boost this person's self-esteem?
4. How can I enable this person to feel loved or give love?

People with dementia sometimes feel unsafe and fearful. They may be anxious or worried about what is happening to them. They may feel out of control. Your help or good intentions may be misunderstood, for example, when you want to give Lucinda a bath or shower. She may appear afraid or agitated for seemingly irrational reasons. In the confused mind of the person with dementia, the situation is threatening. Your role is to interpret Lucinda's unpleasant behavior as an expression of fear. In turn, you are then able to offer safety, comfort, and reassurance through your words and actions.

Many people with dementia don't think of themselves as a person needing care. Their independence is part of their identity, and defines who they are. If Mildred, in the middle stage of dementia, believes that you are taking control and doing something that she is perfectly capable of doing herself, she may express strong disapproval. Instead of using words to express her disapproval, she may resort to pushing, kicking, or other unpleasant responses. An artist of dementia care understands the need to maintain or restore her dignity. Efforts are made to enable her to feel useful and to ensure that she can still do things for herself.

ENVIRONMENTAL REASONS

People with dementia sometimes have difficulty adjusting to their surroundings. The place in which they live may look unfamiliar. There may be too much noise or activity. On the other hand, things may be too quiet—no noise or activity. Navigating the way from one's room to the dining room may seem confusing. The room temperature may be too hot or too cold. Finding a bathroom may seem impossible. The layout, the space, the décor, the walls, the lighting, and all of the things and people in this place—the environment—may trigger challenging behaviors. *Again, stop, look, and listen for potential causes of the behavior.*

The good news is that changes can often be made in the environment to ease or prevent these behaviors. Noise levels can be reduced, room temperatures can be adjusted, stimulating activities can be provided, clutter can be removed, signs and colors can be used as markers, lighting can be improved, and furnishings can be altered to look like a real home.

Consider the following scenario: Lucinda appears to be talking to herself and her tone grows loud and hostile. She is upsetting other residents. You do your best to calm her down but her hostility intensifies. Nothing seems to be triggering Lucinda's increasing agitation. You sit down next to her to watch and listen. You suddenly realize that she is responding to voices she is hearing from a nearby television. Lucinda thinks people are talking to her. However, she cannot fully see or hear the people who are speaking. Failing to get a proper response from the people speaking on the television, Lucinda is angry and upset.

Several things can be tried to calm down Lucinda. You can turn off the television, the source of the voices. You can move Lucinda to an area where the sound from the television is not so loud. You can play some music in the area to muffle the sound from the television. You can ask Lucinda if she would like to wear a headset to listen to her favorite songs on a CD player. It is important to experiment with different ideas until you find one that is successful in reducing disruptive behavior.

THE TRIGGERING TASK

A seemingly simple task like bathing may seem complex and confusing for a person with dementia and trigger a challenging behavior. An activity or task that may appear simple for you may involve a series of steps that the person with dementia can no longer follow in the proper sequence. For example, brushing one's teeth may appear easy to perform but it actually involves a number of specific steps that must be done in proper order to be carried out successfully. Someone like Lucinda may begin a task but then quickly forget how to carry it through to completion. Frustration may grow from repeatedly trying and failing at this task.

The best approach for enabling someone to complete an activity or task is to set the person up for success from the outset. You would not ask someone to solve a complex mathematical problem knowing that the person had limited math skills. People with dementia should be expected to do what they can for as long as possible. But when they reach the point when they do need assistance, they need the support of others such as you. An activity or task may well be accomplished if it is broken down into steps. You may have to offer cues, even one instruction at a time, before moving on to the next step. Encouragement is needed along the way to complete the process.

The following scenario shows how you can be helpful in such situations. Mildred resisted having her clothes changed. Whenever staff approached her, she would pull away and curse. She would begin to kick and grab at anyone who resisted her. However, if a staff member laid out a single item of clothing and politely asked Mildred to try it on, she responded well. She eventually accepted support putting on other items, too.

A powerful way of finding a solution to a challenging behavior is to call upon other staff members for a meeting in a circle. This teamwork can be useful in generating solutions that cannot be imagined alone.

THE SOLUTION CIRCLE

The Solution Circle is a tool for helping you and your colleagues find constructive solutions to difficult behavior. Using a circle to resolve conflict and find creative solutions has its roots in ancient, tribal, and indigenous cultures. Today, the circle is being used successfully in many different ways, such as creating culture change, solving community issues, and reaching creative and innovative solutions to challenges.

The Process

1. Gather together in a circle so that everyone can see each other. There must be no tables or other obstacles in the middle. A circle should consist of no more than twelve people and the exact number of chairs required. There is one important rule—only the person whose turn it is to speak may talk. Everyone else must listen—without comments or questions. (A *speaking wand* may be helpful, such as a flower. The speaker holds the wand to indicate to everyone else "it is my turn." After the first person has responded, the speaking wand is then handed to the next speaker.)
2. The circle starts by one person volunteering to lead that round. The leader then asks for two volunteers: one to

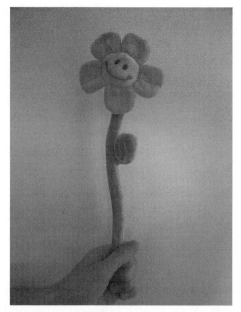

The Speaking Wand.

write down any creative ideas elicited during the circle and the other to be the first to respond to the question.

3. The leader then poses the four questions below—one at a time. The same basic question is asked in different ways. We each tend to favor one of our senses over the others in the ways in which we process information, store it in our memory, and express it. These four questions ensure that every staff member can respond no matter which sense is preferred.

    a. For the *seeing* person: Is there *ever* anyone here who *sees* Mildred in a different light?

    b. For the *hearing* person: Is there *ever* anyone here who *hears* Mildred in a different way?

    c. For the *feeling* person: Is there *ever* anyone here who *feels* differently about Mildred?

    d. For the *thinking* person: Is there *ever* anyone here who *thinks* differently about Mildred?

4. The participants, including the leader, take turns in responding to any of the four questions posed—choosing the one they can best relate to. You can pass if you are not ready to answer. It is the leader's responsibility, once the circle has gone around the first time, to come back to those who passed. A person can pass only once and must therefore respond in the second round.

5. Answers must be of a constructive and positive nature. This is not a time for judgment, ridicule, sarcasm, or skepticism. This session is designed to stimulate creative and positive suggestions.

6. Once *everyone* has taken a turn in responding to the question—and not until then—the circle is open for comments and discussion. The same rule applies that when someone is talking. Everyone else listens.

Through the Solution Circle you will find that the solution lies within your group. It is through intense listening that you learn from your colleagues, and their ideas become an endless source of possibilities.

There may be times when you have tried everything to address the challenging behaviors of your residents, yet nothing seems to work. In spite of your best efforts, you feel powerless and are at a loss for a good solution. Then and only then, is it advisable to introduce a trial dose of medication for a resident who seems uncontrollably agitated or depressed. The person-centered approach, using your social and psychological skills, should always be your first choice as most challenging behaviors can be minimized or resolved in this way.

SUMMARY

An artist of dementia care looks for the reasons behind challenging behaviors. You know and understand that someone who is irritated or aggressive does not intend to cause real harm or hurt. Challenging behaviors are expressions of unmet needs, caused or triggered by

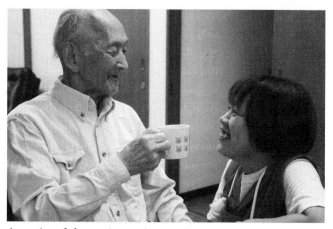

An artist of dementia care knows that a cup of tea, a smile, and a gentle touch create a bond. © Cathy Stein Greenblat

something that makes the person feel threatened, angry, or upset. You look for the underlying physical, social, emotional, and environmental reasons. Once the trigger is identified, it becomes obvious that much can be done to minimize or prevent the challenging behaviors. It takes willpower, creativity, understanding, patience, love, and a desire to do better. As an artist of dementia care, you possess all of these traits and are thereby fully equipped to make life less difficult for people with dementia. More importantly, you can help create the conditions necessary for them to have a good quality of life, too.

THINK ABOUT IT

1. What types of challenging behaviors are most common and what are the most common causes in your experience?
2. Could other interventions carried out by you and other staff members be more effective in overcoming challenging behaviors than psychotropic medications? If yes, describe.
3. Think of a resident who is exhibiting a challenging behavior right now. Have all potential causes been explored? Can you convene a Solution Circle?

5

TAKING CARE OF
FAMILY CAREGIVERS

"Families are like peanut brittle; it takes a whole lot of sugar to keep the nuts together."

—Anonymous

This chapter describes how you can help family caregivers. People with dementia are typically cared for at home by relatives for the major portion of their condition. It is usually many years before the tough decision is made to relocate a loved one to a facility. Family caregivers may include spouses, siblings, in-laws, adult children, grandchildren, and even great-grandchildren. Close friends and neighbors may also be involved in providing care.

These caregivers often have a long personal history with the person with dementia who is now in your care. These caregivers have a deeply rooted interest in making sure that their loved one receives the best possible care from you. They may feel relieved at no longer having to provide constant care at home. On the other hand, they may feel guilty and angry about moving a loved one to a facility or may be suffering the ill effects of long-term caregiving. In addition to the care provided to people with dementia, the artist of dementia care understands that these caregivers often need care too.

Although dementia affects directly one individual, everyone else in that person's social circle is also affected in various ways. Like a pebble cast into a pond, the waves ripple out from the center. Some families work amazingly well together despite the challenges of caregiving, while other families seem filled with tension and conflict. Some individuals within a family make countless sacrifices, yet others do not lift a hand to help. Some family caregivers cope well, while others cope poorly. An artist of dementia care knows that families and individuals respond differently to the challenges of dementia. Some family caregivers desperately need healing and hope to deal with the devastating effects of dementia on loved ones, their families, and themselves, while others can cope with less emotional assistance.

Family caregivers may be pleased by your care and concern but others may be hostile toward you. Caregivers may be accepting of their loved one's dementia but others may be angry, upset, or in denial. Some caregivers may be strong and healthy but others may be fragile, depressed, or exhausted. Some caregivers may offer you praise and compliments but others may offer only complaints. Do not take criticism personally. Their harsh remarks say more about them than anything you have said or done. Family caregivers often suffer emotional pain stemming from guilt and anger. You make a convenient target for what is troubling them. They are hurting inside and their pain is unfortunately expressed in negative words and actions toward others. To better understand and care for family caregivers, let's take a look at the experience of caring for someone with dementia at home.

CARE AT HOME

A national survey of family caregivers by the National Alliance for Caregivers and the Alzheimer's Association showed that a typical individual helping someone with dementia is a woman, 48 years old, married, and employed. She has at least some college education and no children living in the home. The most common caregiving relationship is between a parent and child and one out of six provides care to a grand-parent. Only 6 percent of the caregivers in the survey were spouses; not a surprising figure given that the average age of the care recipient was 78 years old. Most people with dementia live alone or with relatives.

Most caregivers are women and do the majority of the "hands on" work. Two-thirds of caregivers help with one or more personal care tasks such as bathing, feeding, and dealing with incontinence. Fully half of caregivers work full time and two-thirds have missed work because of caregiving responsibilities. Three-quarters of care-givers report unmet needs, such as needing more time for them-selves, help managing stress, and information on managing challeng-ing behaviors. Despite heavy burdens and unmet needs, nearly half of caregivers report having used no paid help in the past 12 months. Nearly a third of caregivers provide care for five years or more.

This same survey also looked at the physical, emotional, social, and financial consequences of caring for relatives with dementia. The survey found:

- 30 percent of caregivers get less exercise than before caregiving.
- 55 percent have less time for other family members.
- 49 percent give up vacations, hobbies, or social activities.
- 41 percent report high levels of emotional stress.
- 20 percent report their health as fair or poor.
- 18 percent say that caregiving has made their health worse.
- 49 percent of non-spouses provide financial assistance.

It is clear that family caregivers confront daily challenges in provid-ing care at home. They often struggle to balance the competing demands of caregiving, work, and other family responsibilities. Mov-ing a loved one to a care facility is often considered a last resort option. There are worries and fears about the quality of care. There is concern about the emotional impact of moving a loved one with dementia who does not adjust well to unfamiliar places and people. Home is considered a safe haven. Nevertheless, many caregivers

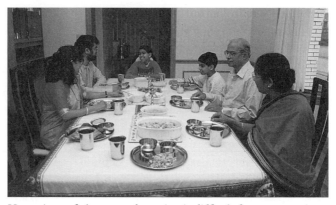

Home is a safe haven and moving is difficult for everyone in the family.

recognize that they cannot continue to provide care 24 hours a day, 7 days a week. Even if other people help out, home care may no longer be viable. An event such as the caregiver's deteriorating health or a loved one's need for more care and supervision may trigger a move to a facility. To many caregivers, this decision represents abandonment of a loved one or a personal failure on their part. A mix of emotions such as sadness, guilt, and anger are likely to be experienced under these difficult circumstances.

LOSS AND GRIEF

Caregivers face a series of losses over the long course of dementia and moving a loved one to a facility represents the most difficult loss. Instead of the normal give-and-take one expects in an adult relationship, dementia slowly results in one person becoming dependent on another person. Recent memories can no longer be shared. Communication becomes strained. Decisions cannot be fully discussed. The relationship they once knew is no longer the same. Managing routine household and personal care tasks may become the focus of the relationship. For spouses, the intimacy of marriage is gradually lost and loneliness may set in. For adult children, the one who parented them gradually needs physical care and emotional support. At the same time, the person with dementia may be physically present yet seem emotionally absent. Not only is the relationship itself threatened, but relationships with others also. Many caregivers report losing friends and becoming socially isolated as they devote more time and energy to a loved one in need.

Caregivers may not appreciate the fact that they are grieving over the many losses and changes they experience as a result of dementia. Grief is a normal reaction to any type of loss, not just death. Caregivers may feel that they have no time to deal with the associated feelings or for grieving over the many losses they experience. However, grief must be addressed if there is to be a healthy adjustment to the losses involved in caring for someone with dementia. Grief involves a psychological workout. Many studies of caregivers describe four phases or steps of grief: denial, anger, letting go, and acceptance.

Denial, according to one dictionary definition, refers to "disbelief in the existence or reality of something." Denial is a common way for caregivers to avoid or lessen the emotional impact of dementia. By denying painful thoughts, feelings, or facts, worry and fear can be prevented or minimized. Statements such as, "Her memory loss is not that bad" or "I know he can help himself; he is just being helpless to spite me" are forms of denial. Rather than accepting the reality of a loved one's mental decline, denial is a way of holding on to the way things used to be in the past. Other signs of denial among caregivers include not seeking a diagnosis and treatment for dementia, refusing to tell others about the situation, failing to ask others for help including not seeking out a facility until it is absolutely necessary.

Let's take a look at denial in the life of Earl, who is in the early stages of dementia:

> Following the death of his wife, Earl's daughter, Emmy, cared for him in his own home and later in her home with the help of her husband and two teen-aged sons. She denied that Earl needed more help and supervision than her family could provide, even after he wandered away from home and wasn't

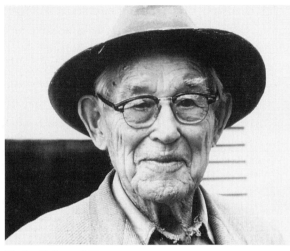

Earl—father of Emmy

found until the next day by the police. When Emmy's marriage and job began to suffer as a result of looking after Earl, she reluctantly agreed to move him to an assisted living facility. Emmy once told her now deceased mother that she would take care of Earl. Emmy believes that this solemn promise has been broken and now she feels terribly guilty.

Let's suppose that the place where Earl now lives is the one in which you work. One day, while Emmy is visiting her father, you overhear her greeting him, "You know who I am, don't you?" You later hear her asking him, "What are the names of your grandchildren?" It is obvious to you that such questions make Earl feel uneasy and set him up for failure. Such questions are clear signs that Emmy is denying the fact that her father no longer has the memory or thinking skills that he once possessed. She is not stupid—she knows that her father has dementia and is forgetful. However, if Earl can somehow remember her or the names of his grandchildren, her guilt might be lessened. On the other hand, if he cannot recall these facts, her guilt may be increased. In either case, Emmy is being unfair to Earl by testing his memory. She is also setting herself up for disappointment if he cannot remember.

Your first reaction may be anger or irritation with Emmy. Rather than expressing these negative feelings to her, what might you say to help her move beyond her state of denial? Some helpful responses might include:

- "I imagine it can be hard at times to have a father with dementia. I also imagine you miss the way he communicated and remembered in the past."
- "Your father is a delightful man with a good sense of humor and warm smile. What was he like before he came to live here?"
- "Is there anything I can do to help make your visits with your father more enjoyable? I have found that he likes to read aloud some of the books that we have on hand."

Rather than reacting to Emmy's questions to her father and aggressively defending Earl, the artist of dementia care responds to Emmy's feelings of hurt and loss. You overcome your initial negative reactions to her and understand that she needs a friend in this difficult time. You reach out to her in a sensitive and caring way. You begin to show her that she can still have a meaningful relationship and rich interactions with her father, despite the profound changes he has experienced due to dementia. You know that it will take more time before she adjusts to his living situation, but your patience will eventually pay off.

Anger is typically the next step in the grief process. Anger is a deep and strong emotion triggered when denial gives way to the painful reality of loss. Anger may be directed toward the person with dementia, oneself, other relatives, friends, staff members, or God. Anger involves facing up to the fact that life is no longer the same. Statements such as, "These staff members don't do a thing to help!" or "What did I do to deserve this?" are signs of anger. Although anger is often expressed to others in words and actions, it can also get bottled up inside oneself resulting in depression. In either case, it becomes obvious to other people that a caregiver's emotions are running high.

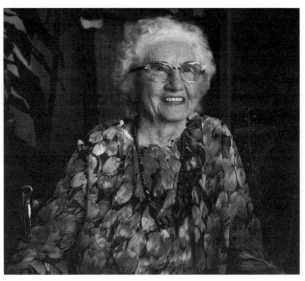

Mildred is married to Martin, but she can no longer remember him.

Anger and depression may become destructive and ruin relationships with others unless a caregiver moves beyond these feelings.

Let's turn to how anger is expressed by Martin, the husband of Mildred, who is in the middle stages of dementia. Martin and Mildred have been married for 56 years. Unfortunately, Mildred cannot recall that they are married. Martin cared for her at home for about eight years until his worsening heart condition made it impossible to continue to care for her at home. Although no longer in denial about the need for Mildred to live in a care facility, Martin does not like the arrangement. In fact, he hates it, although his deep feelings are rooted in his grief over losing his wife to dementia and his resulting loneliness. Unfortunately, Martin tends to express his anger toward staff members. He seems to go out of his way to complain and find fault with others. He speaks harshly to direct care staff, their supervisors, and the administrator. Everyone in the facility dreads the time of day when he visits Mildred because they know to expect trouble.

One day Martin arrives in Mildred's room. He searches frantically for her favorite sweater but it is missing. He says to the staff member assigned to Mildred in a loud voice, "Where the hell is her sweater? I want it found and returned immediately. You people can't get anything right. I should call the police and report a theft!" When the staff member responds in a defensive way, Martin says, "I'm sick of all the excuses. I am going to tell the administrator that you and all of the other fools around here should be fired." His angry outburst appears to upset other residents, including Mildred. Quite naturally, the staff member feels embarrassed and demeaned by this verbal assault. It is difficult not to react angrily to Martin, whose hostility is readily apparent. What might you say to him to address his anger in a constructive way? Some helpful responses might include:

- "You have a legitimate complaint. I am sorry that you are so upset. Talking to my supervisor or the administrator in a quiet place might be the best thing you can do right now."
- "I can understand that you are angry that Mildred's sweater is missing. You are a good husband in the way that you protect her and her belongings. However, I ask you not to take your anger out on me. Just like you, I want Mildred to keep her nice things too."
- "I am sorry that Mildred's sweater is missing. I will do everything I can to find it. Right now, I am also concerned about you. I can appreciate that you are angry and upset."

There is no guarantee that Martin will respond well to any of these statements. However, the artist of dementia care sees through his anger and understands that the sweater is not what is at stake. Martin is hurting and angry. Sadly, Mildred treats him like a stranger. When you acknowledge his anger and direct his attention to solving the problem of the missing sweater, you let him know that you care. After all, you are there for both Mildred and him. As a matter of fact, caring for Martin may be more challenging than caring for Mildred! Someone like Martin who is truly troubled needs much more help than you alone can provide. His anger must be addressed through a team effort and perhaps other forms of help, such as a support group or professional counseling. However, you can be compassionate toward him without enabling him to treat you like a doormat.

The next phase in the grief process is referred to as "letting go." This occurs when a caregiver's anger gives way to realistic expectations about a loved one with dementia. Despite one's best efforts, dementia will not go away. Being angry is a natural reaction but it will not resolve the problem and may make things worse. Blaming oneself or others does not work. There is a gradual realization that a new way of thinking about the situation is required. At this point, a caregiver is still unsure what type of new relationship with a loved one with dementia is possible but certainly the old relationship is not the same anymore. A caregiver begins to let go of hope for the way life used to be. Instead of longing for the past, there is a growing sense that a new kind of "normal" is possible. The doom and gloom of anger and depression may slowly be replaced with hope for a brighter tomorrow.

Let's examine "letting go" in the case of Lucas, the son of Lucinda, who is in the late stages of dementia. Lucas had been very angry that his sister did not "do right" by their mother when she moved Lucinda into your facility. Although Lucas' sister had cared for Lucinda in her home for many years, Lucas did not give his sister proper credit for her hard work and sacrifices. In fact, he caused a rift in the family by casting blaming and guilt at his sister. He seldom visits Lucinda and when he does visit, he usually interacts with her briefly and leaves in a hurry.

One day while Lucas is visiting his mother, you notice him trying in vain to engage her in a conversation. She can no longer comprehend what he is saying and has lost most of her speech. Lucinda looks at him blankly. He turns to you and says, "I can't even talk to my mother any more. No wonder my sister put her in here. How can you do this kind of work all the time?"

There is still a hint of anger in Lucas, but he is beginning to understand her reasons for moving her to your facility. Caring for Lucinda at home became too painful and he is now experiencing

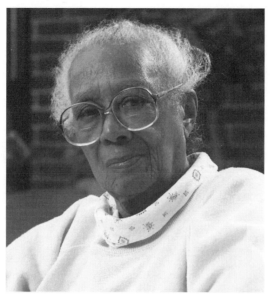

Lucinda—mother of Lucas who grieves over
the mother he once knew and loved.

some of that pain. Rather than blaming his sister, he is now trying to
accept his sister's decision. He is questioning his old way of thinking
and appears to be looking for a new course. At the same time, he
thinks that his relationship with his mother is finished. He does not
know what an artist of dementia care knows—that there are ways
to communicate with Lucinda other than through talking. Here are
some suggested responses to Lucas:

- "I imagine it is hard for you and your sister to see your
  mother living here. But she is in good hands. We love
  spending time with her and she is pleasant and content.
  When I sing a tune, she often joins in by humming or
  singing. Shall we try it with her together?"
- "You and your sister both want what is best for your
  mother. I really enjoy taking care of her and she often
  winks and smiles back at me. I try to see what's left of each

person instead of thinking about what they can no longer do. Your mother is still very much alive."

- "You and your sister must love your mother very much. Although she seems far away at times, Lucinda is really quite present in the moment. I can show you how well she responds when music is played."

Such statements may enable Lucas to support his sister's decision. They may also enable him to change his behavior toward his mother. Rather than thinking that his relationship with her has ended, perhaps he can make adjustments to the changes that have happened. Rather than lament over how much Lucinda has changed due to dementia, perhaps he can still connect with her in meaningful ways by changing his own behavior and attitudes. The artist of dementia care can lead Lucas forward as he searches for a new way of relating to his mother. What you have learned with time and experience, you can pass along to others.

The final phase of grief is acceptance. This happens when the task of letting go is complete. It involves a sense of gratitude for all that has happened in spite of the many challenges. There is no longer a preoccupation with the past or regrets about what might have been. The focus is now on the present as well as the future. Participation in new activities and relationships beyond the role of caregiver become possible.

A woman who cared for her husband put it this way: "I learned to be a strong woman because of my husband's illness. I would not wish Alzheimer's disease on anybody but it taught me a lot about myself. I loved my husband more than I could have imagined and he gave me a confidence in myself that nobody can ever take away."

In her memoir *Mom, Are You Still There?* Kathleen Negri describes her anger about her mother's illness and conflicts with her father and her siblings over care decisions. However, she writes of her eventual acceptance of the situation:

"I finally recognized that I could not control anything or anyone except myself to make this a rewarding and constructive process for me. I came back to myself, where I had the opportunity to become empowered; to fashion my own reality about dementia. And, it was here, by focusing my attention on myself and my thoughts, and by giving myself permission to feel everything—all my healthy and unhealthy emotions—I grew better equipped to accompany my mother on her journey through Alzheimer's. It was here that I found a path of love and compassion."

Caregivers do not pass through these phases of grief in one fell swoop. There are far too many losses in the course of dementia to reach acceptance, once and for all. The series of losses and accompanying grief is why caregivers often describe a sense of riding an emotional roller coaster—a winding road of ups and downs.

Sadly, some people never accept their loved one's dementia, the move to a care facility, or the involvement of other caregivers like you. Sometimes they reach acceptance only after the death of their relative with dementia. Unfortunately, they get bogged down in anger and resentment and are ongoing sources of irritation for other people. Having a close friend, a professional counselor, or a support group along for this difficult journey may help them to reach acceptance. You can play a small but important role in this healing process as well.

The artist of dementia care recognizes that everyone grieves in their own way and at their own pace. The best you can do is to validate that the changes are difficult for them and hopefully they will find some measure of peace along this challenging, personal journey. You can give them that great hope whenever they come for a visit.

MAKING THE MOST OF VISITS

You may encounter families at care conferences or other meetings, but perhaps the most valuable time to interact with them is when they are visiting their relatives in your facility. Many family caregivers

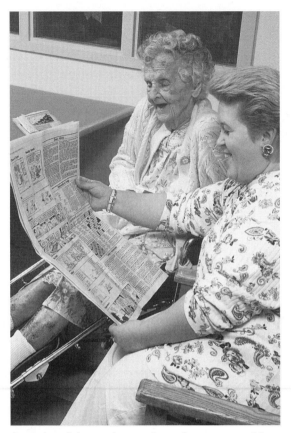

An artist of dementia care shows how to turn visits
into meaningful moments.

struggle to have pleasurable visits but you are in a position to teach
them. You can tell them that it is usually overwhelming for someone
with dementia to have too many visitors at once; visits by one or two
people are likely to be more enjoyable than visits involving three or
more people. You can also tell them that visits can be kept short,
keeping in mind that the quality of time is more important than the
quantity of time. You can also give them simple ideas to make visits
pleasurable.

The artist of dementia care knows how to have meaningful interactions with someone with dementia. You know how to communicate in a variety of ways, not just words. Our culture tends to view social interactions in terms of conversation. This puts limits on visiting someone with dementia. Family caregivers often do not know what to do or say. Visits are more satisfying if they are activity based—doing something together. It is best to engage in activities that combine some or all of the five senses, including seeing, hearing, smelling, touching, and tasting. Of course, activities must be suited to the needs, preferences, and abilities of each person with dementia. However, most activities can be adapted for people at any stage. Here are some simple one-to-one activities that you might introduce to family caregivers:

- Holding hands while listening to music
- Singing favorite tunes or hymns
- Looking at old photos
- Making scrapbooks
- Baking cookies
- Tending to plants
- Watching and feeding the birds
- Attending to personal care such as polishing nails or using cosmetics
- Sharing a "read-aloud" book such as *The Sunshine on My Face* by Lydia Burdick. *Happy New Year to You!* by Lydia Burdick and Jane Freeman or the four-part series by Patricia Garbarini including *Spring in the Park, Summer by the Water, Autumn in the Country,* and *Winter Fun*
- Reciting familiar prayers
- Performing household tasks such as laundry, cleaning a room, or setting a table
- Interacting with dolls
- Drawing or painting pictures
- Walking in a garden

- Watching a nature program on television, DVD or video
- Dancing
- Playing a simple game
- Patting animals, such as dogs and cats
- Sharing or assisting with a meal
- Exercising
- Putting together a simple jigsaw puzzle
- Doing a handicraft
- Smelling perfumes or aromatic oils such as lavender, rose, orange, lemon, and frankincense
- Massaging the body with creams and lotions

The key to a successful visit is to be prepared with a simple activity. It may be helpful to have "activity boxes" available with the tools necessary to carry out the above activities. Ask your Activity Director to assemble some things that could be easily used by both you and visitors. Remind family caregivers that the goal is not to do something productive or to have a concrete outcome. The true purpose of a visit is seen in the process of doing something together and connecting joyfully through rich interactions in the present moment. Young children, free of inhibitions, know how to do this naturally. They are experts in fun and spontaneity. Whenever possible, they should be called upon to take part in visits. Besides, most people with dementia "light up" in the company of young children, especially toddlers and babies.

TAKING CARE OF YOU

An African proverb tells us, "It takes a village to raise a child." Many people are likewise needed to care for someone with dementia as well as their family caregivers. The work you do cannot be done alone. You may have a big heart, plus lots of experience and expertise, but you also need and deserve a support system. You naturally become attached to your residents. When they decline and die it is normal to feel sad. Who picks you up when you are down? Remember that you are part of a team. If the members of your team are not working well together, be sure to find a friend in whom you can confide your thoughts and feelings. The artist of dementia care seeks out others for mutual support.

Whenever you board an airplane, the flight attendant announces before take off that oxygen masks will drop from the ceiling in the event of an emergency. You are instructed to first put on your own mask or else you run the risk of not having enough oxygen to help others. Likewise, your first obligation is to make sure that you remain healthy—physically, emotionally, and spiritually. It is not selfish to practice self-care. It is indeed a necessity in order to stay fresh and focused on being an artist of dementia care. Eating properly, getting enough sleep, taking breaks, praying, listening to music, watching movies, dancing, and singing are just a few examples. Decide what works best for you and then routinely practice self-care.

It takes a strong person to recognize that everyone has limits. All of us need help from others from time to time. Your residents demonstrate this important lesson about the human condition every single day. Only by caring for yourself can you continue to care for others in loving ways. The artist of dementia care understands the connection between caring for oneself and caring for others.

THINK ABOUT IT

1. What do family members need from you most of all when they move their relative with dementia into your facility?
2. Think about a particularly challenging family member of one of your residents. Where do think this person may be in the grief process described above? What might be done to help this family caregiver?

3. List one active step you can take in the next week to care for yourself. What specifically do you want to do for yourself and when do you plan to do it? On a scale of 1 to 10, with 10 as the highest score, what is your confidence level in achieving this plan? If less than a 7, revise the active step to make it more achievable. Write down your plan; share it with another person and assess your progress in one week. Keep up this plan by adding new ways of caring for yourself each week.

Chapter

THE ARTIST IN ACTION

". . . a man does not consist of memory alone. He has feelings, will, sensibilities, is a moral being . . . and it is here that you can find a way to touch him. In the realm of the individual, there is much that you can do."

—A.R. Luria,
Russian psychologist

How do you know when the art of dementia care is being put into action? What does an artist do differently than other staff members? In this final chapter, many examples highlight both the art and the artist. The positive behaviors and attitudes of the artist who provides person-centered care are contrasted with the behaviors and attitudes of the non-artist. These differences will better define your role and responsibilities in providing the best possible care for your residents with dementia.

The artist of dementia care makes a conscious effort to continuously treat residents in a person-centered fashion, whereas the non-artist does not do so consistently. The non-artist provides just the basics to those with dementia—keeping them safe, clean, and fed. This level of care meets minimum standards to provide for the physical well-being of residents. It is important to accomplish these physical care tasks. In fact, on those days when your facility is short staffed, performing this basic level of care may require a heroic effort on your part. However, the artist of dementia care goes beyond providing good physical care and strives to promote other aspects of residents' well-being: mental, social, emotional, and spiritual. Treating everyone with dementia as whole persons contributes to their quality of life. At the same time, the artist becomes a role model for co-workers and assures family members that their loved one is in the best hands. You can feel good about the positive impact you have on everyone, especially your residents.

PUTDOWNS AND UPLIFTS

Dr. Tom Kitwood, mentioned earlier, was a leading advocate in a movement to recognize the humanity of people with dementia. Based on close observations of people with dementia living in care facilities, he described 17 attitudes and behaviors that diminish their humanity. He called them "personal detractors"—small acts that detract or take away the self-esteem of people with dementia. When personal detractors are carried out, they diminish the well-being of people with dementia and often trigger disturbing responses in them.

We refer here to personal detractors as "putdowns." In other words, putdowns are attitudes and behaviors that dehumanize or diminish someone; although they are seldom done deliberately to cause personal harm. These acts are typically carried out in an unthinking or unconscious manner, without regard for the effects on people with dementia. Putdowns are behaviors and attitudes that fail to honor the individuality of residents. An artist of dementia care works hard to counter such putdowns by relating to people with dementia in ways that uphold their well-being.

The opposite of "putdowns" are what we call "uplifts." These are positive or uplifting attitudes and behaviors that create rich interactions between you and your residents. Uplifts are conscious acts of kindness, care, and concern. They represent the best aspects of person-centered care. When practiced continuously, uplifts reinforce well-being—your own, and those in your care. A good quality of life becomes a reality for all concerned.

In this chapter, we contrast 17 putdowns with 17 uplifts. The artist of dementia care strives at all times to work toward making uplifts a way of life for all residents. You might think that the putdowns described here are too extreme and are rarely experienced by your residents. However, they are based on real life experiences and subtle forms of putdowns routinely occur. It is remarkably easy to slip into the attitudes and behaviors of putdowns, especially if other staff members use them regularly or you are tired and stressed.

It takes a conscious effort to become an artist of dementia care and consistently enact uplifts among people with dementia. If you practice them, you create the right conditions for them to experience well-being and reduce the risk of challenging behaviors. You can take satisfaction in knowing that your residents live in a place where they are loved, respected, and truly thrive.

To *Intimidate versus to* Empathize

Intimidation is a putdown that refers to making someone fearful through threats, coercion, or physical power. For example, Mildred is seen putting on a necklace that belongs to another resident. The staff member who sees this happen says to Mildred, in an accusing voice, "If you don't stop touching that necklace, you will be in big trouble. You had better put it down!" Due to fear and the threat of punishment, Mildred will likely remove the necklace immediately. However, she will have been intimidated and devalued. Perhaps she thought that the necklace was her own and was merely trying on what she thought belonged to her. She may feel misunderstood, fearful, or even angry about the harsh reaction.

In contrast to intimidation, the artist of dementia care empathizes with Mildred by seeing the situation from her point of view. Instead of accusing and instigating a problem, it is understood that Mildred is putting on the necklace for a valid reason. She is respected without

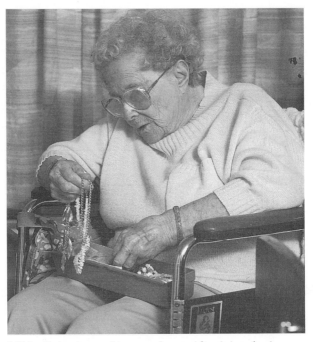

Mildred's joy in touching another resident's jewelry is an act of pleasure, not theft.

judgment. The artist understands that Mildred means no harm; she is simply fulfilling an unmet need—perhaps to feel beautiful—by trying on a necklace. An uplifting response in this situation might be, "Mildred, you look beautiful in Betty's necklace. Let's find Betty and ask her if you can borrow the necklace for a while. Is that a good idea?"

To Withhold versus to Be Compassionate

Withholding involves refusing to give attention that is requested by someone with dementia or not meeting an obvious need. Withholding may seem justified at times, especially if someone repeatedly asks for help. For example, Lucinda is sitting in a wheelchair and crying out, "Help me! Help me! Help me!" It is obvious that Lucinda is distressed. A staff member declares, "There she goes again—always seeking attention!" The staff member chooses to withhold attention from Lucinda based on her habit of calling out for help. It makes no difference why she is asking for help.

In contrast to withholding help, an artist accepts her plea at face value and responds compassionately. The focus is put on Lucinda and not just on her behavior. It is understood that she is calling out because she has a need that has not been met. Perhaps she is hungry, thirsty, lonely, or in pain. A compassionate artist finds out what is bothering Lucinda instead of dismissing her. The uplifting artist might greet Lucinda warmly, give her a hug, and say to her in a soothing voice, "Lucinda, what can I do for you right now?"

To Accuse versus to Understand

An *accusation* is a putdown in which someone with dementia is blamed for actions or failures of actions that arise from his or her disability. For example, Lucinda is seen taking some food from another resident's plate and a staff member says, "Stop stealing Ron's food. Put it down. You know it doesn't belong to you!" In fact, Lucinda does not know the difference between her plate and another resident's plate. She may be hungry, and without her usual social inhibitions, she may simply grab the food to satisfy her hunger. Having been put down by the insensitive staff member, she may withdraw or become upset.

An artist of dementia care understands that there is a reason for Lucinda's behavior. It is senseless to accuse her of anything. Instead, understanding is called for in this instance, such as, "Lucinda, I can see that you are hungry. May I offer you some food right now? Today, do you prefer chicken or fish?"

To Invalidate versus to Validate

Invalidation means to reject the perspective of people with dementia or to negate their opinions. For example, let's say Earl is a new resident in your facility. He is not settling in very well and he repeatedly says in a loud voice, "I want to go home! I don't belong here. Will someone please take me home?" An inexperienced or well-meaning staff member might reply to Earl, "Don't worry. This is your home now. You will get used to it." Although this reply is an attempt to pacify Earl, it does not address his underlying feelings. In fact, it ignores his entire experience and the need behind his expression. He feels out of sorts, but nobody is responding to his confused state.

Instead of disregarding Earl's desire to go home, the artist knows that he is really feeling afraid or lonely. He feels like a stranger in this unfamiliar place and needs to feel comfortable. In a genuine, warm, caring voice he could be asked, "Earl, are you looking for someone? Can I introduce you to the other people here? We have some wonderful folks I'd like you to meet."

To Infantilize versus to Honor

Infantilization means to treat a person with dementia in a patronizing or condescending manner, as an insensitive parent might treat a young child. Such an attitude or behavior disregards the age and

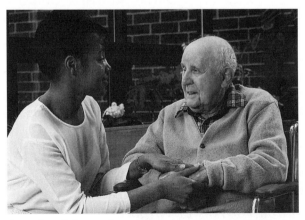

An artist of dementia care focuses on the emotional needs of people who have dementia rather than how those needs are expressed.

experience of the residents. For example, Earl is seen urinating inside a closet. A staff member reacts with sharp disapproval, "Earl, you naughty boy! Look at the mess you have made! Don't ever do that again! I should make you clean that up."

In contrast, an artist of dementia care immediately recognizes that Earl probably felt he had no choice and did what seemed natural to him at the time. Instead of drawing attention to his unpleasant behavior, he is simply redirected without judgment and asked, "Earl, may I direct you to the bathroom?" Every effort is made to preserve his dignity instead of causing him any embarrassment. The closet is cleaned up without complaint and staff members are asked to look for any signs in the future that Earl needs to use the bathroom. An artist asks oneself, "How might I prevent this incident from happening again?"

To Objectify versus to Personalize

Objectification refers to treating someone like an object instead of as a person. There is little or no regard for one's feelings. For example, Mildred is chatting with other residents when a staff member suddenly places a blood pressure cuff on her arm. Conversation stops as the staff member goes about taking Mildred's blood pressure. No regard is shown for Mildred or the other residents who are present and the conversation they were involved in. Their personal space is invaded without explanation. In another example, a staff member pushes Earl away in his wheelchair without permission. He is startled and has been given no say in the matter. In either case, Mildred and Earl were unwilling participants in the hurried activity of insensitive staff members.

An artist recognizes that Mildred is a person deserving of respect and dignity. In contrast to treating her like an object, she is uplifted when asked for her permission to do things both *with* her and *for* her. Mildred appreciates it when you approach her from the front and make eye contact with her, "Excuse me Mildred. I would like to make sure that your blood pressure is okay. Can I place this cuff around your arm to check your blood pressure?" In the case of Earl, a personalized encounter would begin with a similar request, "Hello Earl. I would like to invite you to the dining room for dinner. May I push you there in your wheelchair?"

To Mock versus to Pay Respect

Mockery refers to the humiliating practice of making fun of someone. Fortunately, mocking someone with dementia is rare but when it happens, it is a sure sign that a staff member has lost a caring attitude. For example, Lucinda repetitively makes the sound, "Ooh! Ooh! Ooh!" In response, a staff member mimics her, laughs aloud, and says to her, "You sound like an old foghorn!" Lucinda is mocked for her inability to express herself in a "normal" way. She has been insulted, whether or not she understands the meaning of the words.

An artist of dementia care would never disrespect someone with dementia. Each person is worthy of respect regardless of one's capacity for memory, thinking, or language. An artist uplifts Lucinda by understanding what it is she is trying to communicate. An artist uses empathy and intuition to find out what is bothering her, "Lucinda, it sounds like you are trying to tell me something. Are you in pain? Are you sad? How can I help you?"

To Stigmatize versus to Affirm

A stigma refers to a mark of shame or disgrace. *Stigmatization* involves treating people with dementia as if they deserve to be outcasts. For example, Lucinda has been gibbering for the past ten minutes and a staff member remarks to another one as a birthday party is about to begin, "Don't bother with that one! She's got nothing left in her head. You can let her be." In other words, a decision is reached that Lucinda is too impaired to enjoy the birthday party. The staff member thinks she can be excluded from the party.

Rather than setting people with dementia apart for what they lack, an artist of dementia care affirms everyone's humanity and acknowledges Lucinda's needs, even though she is unable to speak up in customary ways. An artist makes every effort to include her in appropriate activities and encourages others to do the same. Lucinda's self-esteem is improved when she is accepted for the way she is. An artist might say, "Lucinda, may I invite you to join me at the birthday party? I would love to have you there as my guest."

To Ignore versus to Acknowledge

Ignoring refers to situations in which staff members carry on a conversation or activity as if people with dementia are not present. For example, two staff members talk with each other while one assists Mildred with her meal. They have a private conversation as if Mildred does not exist. The role of assisting Mildred to eat is neither important to them nor do they believe it is necessary to include her in their conversation. After all, they apparently believe that she can be ignored.

To acknowledge Mildred, on the other hand, means that her presence is recognized. As an artist of dementia care, you focus your attention solely on Mildred and include her in your conversations and activities. You know that Mildred is easily distracted by conversation during mealtime and needs peace and quiet while being assisted with her meal. When you talk, you talk directly to her and nobody else.

To Disempower versus to Empower

Disempowerment involves preventing a person with dementia from using his or her remaining abilities or failing to help him or her to complete actions that they may initiate. Disempowerment means to intervene and take over when unnecessary. It promotes dependence on others and fosters a sense of helplessness. For example, a staff member might take over dressing Mildred although she might be able to complete some or all parts of this task for herself if given some time and encouragement. Although it might be quicker to dress Mildred without her input, she is indirectly being told by this action that she has lost the ability to dress herself. She has lost control over her life, even in the most intimate details such as dressing. She may react with hostility, especially if she is accustomed to having a say in matters that affect her.

To empower someone with dementia means to promote independence and the use of one's abilities. There is no question in the previous example that Mildred needs some level of support. The important question is how much support she really needs. An artist of dementia care looks for opportunities to involve Mildred as much as possible and give her some control over her life. Opportunities are given to encourage her to share as fully as possible in her care and decisions affecting her. In this case, she could be assisted in picking out her clothes, laying them out on her bed, and talking her through the steps of putting on each piece of clothing. This process can appear time consuming. However, the artist knows that Mildred feels empowered and successful when she dresses herself. Coaching and coaxing her through the steps of dressing will pay off when she smiles as she looks in the mirror.

To Disparage versus to Boost Self-esteem

Disparagement means to tell someone that he or she is incompetent, useless, or worthless. This usually occurs in subtle forms. For example, Mildred offers to do the dishes after breakfast but she is told, "No, thank you. You just sit back and relax. You have done enough dishes in your life. We'll do them now!" A more glaring example of this putdown is seen when a staff member says, "Earl, let me finish tying your shoe laces. You know you can't do that for yourself!" The actions of these staff members remind both Mildred and Earl that they are incapable of contributing in meaningful ways. Their self-esteem has been further diminished.

In contrast, an artist of dementia care looks for different ways to engage residents to enable them to feel needed or useful. Although they might lack the initiative to offer any help, they often desperately want to feel needed and useful. An artist knows that they simply need to be asked. They will almost always respond to invitations to do things that they can still do well or with minimal assistance. For example, you could ask, "Mildred, I need a hand. Would you be able to help me do the dishes?" You may choose part of an activity that you know she can perform successfully and praise her for her contribution. Through your invitation and her active participation, Mildred's self-esteem will be boosted.

In the case of Earl trying to tie his shoelaces, you might patiently watch him but do not interfere unless he appears frustrated. Then, and only then, would you kindly suggest, "What if I give you a hand with those shoelaces, Earl? They look like they are being difficult." Instead of rushing to his aid and taking over for him, you coach him along so he makes a contribution to his own care.

To Deceive versus to Support

Deception refers to manipulating or taking advantage of someone with dementia due to impairments in memory and judgment. This includes telling outright lies or "therapeutic fibs." Such practices may make things easier for a short while but they undermine self-esteem and well-being. For example, Lucinda's daughter has just left the care facility and now Lucinda is crying. A staff member attempts to reassure Lucinda by saying, "No need to feel upset. Your daughter has just stepped away for a minute and will return soon." Although well meaning, the statement is not true and does not address Lucinda's emotional needs. The false statement is aimed at getting her to quiet down and shows no regard for her upset feelings.

On the other hand, to be supportive means to share in the moment with someone with dementia and accept his or her feelings. The feelings and needs of the person are always priorities for an artist of dementia care. You attempt to understand and address feelings or needs based upon what you know about the person as an individual. In this instance, you might give Lucinda a hug and in a caring tone of voice say, "I know you are upset when your daughter leaves. I am sorry that you are sad. What if we make a cup of tea? Then we can sit and have a nice talk and you can tell me all about your daughter." In this way, Lucinda's feelings are acknowledged and she feels supported. At the same time, she can form a bond with you and take part in a pleasurable activity.

To Impose versus to Promote Autonomy

Imposition refers to forcing someone with dementia to do something without one's consent. In a less subtle form, it can also mean denying someone the possibility of choice. For example, a staff member is focused on the task of getting Mildred dressed and says to her,

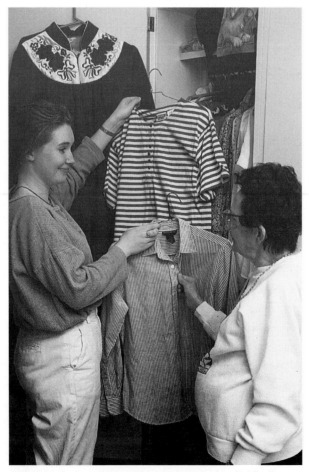

Offering choice promotes autonomy and individuality.

"Here is the shirt that you are going to wear today." Mildred is left with no choice in the matter. She is reminded that she has no power and must accept someone else's authority.

In contrast, an artist of dementia care recognizes personal preferences and offers choices, no matter how small. Opportunities are provided to exercise control over decisions. For example, Mildred could be shown two shirts and asked, "Today, are you going to wear the striped shirt or the blue one?" Although she has just two choices, the final decision is left to her.

To Label versus to Describe

The problem of labeling people with dementia has already been addressed, but it is worth reviewing. Again, labeling refers to a type of shorthand language used to categorize others and their experience with words such as *Demented, Wanderer, Feeder, Screamer,* or *Sundowner.* These labels reduce people to their symptoms or impairments rather than respecting them as full human beings separate from their impairments. For example, a staff member announces, "Let's get all the sundowners like Mildred involved in an activity before they start acting out." Mildred and the others are grouped together and labeled as problems rather than seen as individual people.

In contrast, an artist of dementia care avoids labels and always treats people as unique individuals. Behaviors and attitudes are carefully described in ways that respect each person. You might say, "Before Mildred feels restless today, I would like to invite her and others to the lounge where we can sing and dance together."

To Disrupt versus to Stand Back

Disruption refers to suddenly intrude upon or interrupt someone with dementia. In such instances, staff members put their own agendas ahead of the needs of the resident. For example, several residents, including Earl, are playing a board game with a staff member when another staff member disrupts the group and declares loudly, "It's time for Earl to have his bath! Come with me Earl." It is as if Earl's activity is completely unimportant and the rest of the group are invisible. Everyone is put down in this scenario, especially Earl, who is singled out.

On the other hand, an artist of dementia care stands back and waits for an appropriate time to intervene. The resident is afforded the courtesy of being able to take part in an activity without interruption. An artist would patiently wait until the group activity had ended and then quietly ask, "Are you ready for a warm bath, Earl?" Alternatively, Earl might have his bath before the group meets for a board game.

To Banish versus to Include

Banishment is a putdown that involves excluding or sending someone away. It means separating and isolating someone with dementia from others. For example, Lucinda is having a bad day and repeatedly spits out her food at lunch while sitting with three other residents. In exasperation, a staff member removes her from the dining room. Lucinda is taken to her room without any food. She is treated as a naughty child who is being told off. Even though she is unable to complain due to language problems, Lucinda may feel rejected.

In contrast, an artist of dementia care always seeks to include the person. You sit alongside and involve the resident whose behavior is upsetting you or others. In Lucinda's case, you would find out the reason she is spitting out her food. If nothing seems to work, you would invite her to have her meal with you at another table. Lucinda might also be left alone for a short time in order for her to calm down, but she would not be ignored or left on her own as a punishment. She would be shown genuine respect and know that she still belongs in spite of her difficulty eating that day.

To Outpace versus to Pace

Outpacing is perhaps the most common putdown of all. It involves providing information or presenting choices at a rate too fast for a person to understand. It may also involve putting pressure on someone to do things more rapidly than tolerated.

A staff member might say in a hurried voice to Mildred, "You are going to the beauty shop this morning. Do you want your bath beforehand or afterward? You can do it at either time but it would be helpful to know right away. What do you think?" Mildred becomes overwhelmed by this quick and confusing information. She cannot remember it, understand it, or make a decision.

An artist of dementia care, on the other hand, recognizes the slowed abilities of people with dementia and adapts one's pace of speech accordingly. It's similar to walking slowly alongside someone using crutches. You deliberately slow your pace to match the speed or ability of the other person. To keep things simple for Mildred, you might say, "Good morning, Mildred. Would you prefer a bath now or later today?" This is an easy question for her to understand and answer.

CONCLUSION

When you practice the art of dementia care, providing *great* care is your aim. You must learn to think on your feet and make snap decisions. You can respond compassionately to any challenge you may face because you have the confidence and experience to make a positive difference in the lives of people with dementia. Their disabilities are challenging at times, but you are committed to finding creative solutions to meet their needs. You learn how to enter into their world and see through their eyes and listen with their ears. You create a positive environment in which people with dementia can feel safe, and close to other people. They truly feel at home.

You play a critical role in contributing to the well-being of people with dementia. Your work has meaning and purpose beyond anything you can imagine. You have the power to bring joy and happiness into their lives at a time when they need it the most. Your words or actions can put them down or lift them up. An artist of dementia care strives to eliminate putdowns and continuously practices uplifts. You take responsibility for enriching the lives of everyone in your care and creating a loving home.

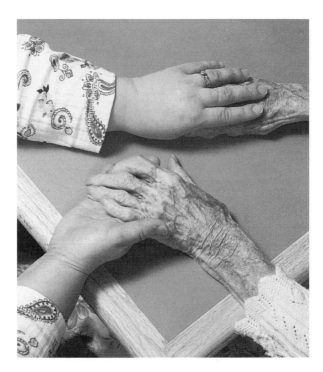

THINK ABOUT IT

1. As you read the descriptions of the 17 putdowns and uplifts, which ones have you noticed recently in your facility? How can you work to reduce and eventually eliminate putdowns and replace them with uplifts?
2. Think of a person with dementia in your facility who seems disliked or ignored by other residents or staff. Describe three uplifts that might be tried with this person.
3. How might the staff at your facility relate to one another if uplifts were commonplace?

A VIEW FROM THE FIELD

The following examples are derived from actual experiences.

THE SHARK

At mealtimes, Rose drove all the other residents crazy by circling the tables while everyone else was dining. Staff members had tried numerous ways to get her to sit down with no success. All they achieved was that Rose would become angry and tell them to go away. Staff members began to refer to Rose by an unflattering nickname, the shark.

Unmet Need: *To feel needed and useful*

On looking back into her history, a staff member discovered that Rose had been a waitress during her working years; so, naturally, she could not sit down while others were eating. She was now recreating a time when she was needed and useful and had an identity.

Solution

Rose was given an apron and treated as a staff member. Staff provided her with a cart that she could wheel around and pick up plates, cups, and utensils at the dining tables after each meal. She waited anxiously for other residents to finish eating so she could spring into action. When she completed making her rounds of the tables, she was accompanied to the kitchen where she unloaded everything. Staff made a special effort to thank her at the end of each meal. Rose rarely dropped anything and was all smiles whenever she put on the apron. On her birthday, the administrator gave Rose a special apron with her name imprinted and she was also recognized with a plaque for her service.

KILLING THE JOY

Every time it came to having fun in a group activity, Dulcie clammed up and became sad, depressed, and upset. No matter how staff members tried to encourage her to join in, she refused to take part in any frivolity.

Unmet Need: *To feel safe in expressing joy and pleasure*

A staff member looking into Dulcie's childhood wondered if perhaps she had not been allowed to have fun and asked, "Were you not allowed to be happy when you were little?"

With little prompting, Dulcie opened up and began to tell stories of how her parents would often scold her. If she came home with tadpoles, she was reprimanded and told to throw them out. If she danced, she was told to stop until, eventually, all the joy was punished out of her.

Solution

In this situation, the solution was simple. All that was needed was for staff members to truly validate Dulcie as a person who was allowed to express joy by reiterating, "Here it's okay to have fun. Here it is safe." After a short time, Dulcie began to join in and now it seems she is making up for lost time with her ready smile and frequent laughter.

QUALITY CONTROLLER

Harold became unpopular with his fellow residents because he continually visited their rooms, uninvited, and would check their bedding. Pulling back the cover and untucking the blankets, he would run his hands over the material then walk away leaving the bed unmade and the occupant infuriated. Great frustration and anger grew towards Harold from the residents, and staff members were increasingly upset with no idea what to do.

Unmet Need: *To feel needed and useful*

Staff members checked into his background and learned that Harold had actually designed a special blanket during his career at a textile factory. He had worked with fabrics and bedding materials in particular. Material and textiles had been his life. Now, he was not deliberately messing up other residents' beds, but merely checking the quality, fabric, and texture of the covers in an attempt to regain his identity and feel useful again.

Solution

Staff members accepted the suggestion to provide laundry for Harold to fold, and beds for him to make up. He was given opportunities to be in contact with familiar materials and to do real, meaningful jobs, which in turn boosted his self-esteem. After a short time, Harold ceased visiting other residents' rooms except to say hello.

HERDING THE CATTLE

Staff members and residents were tearing their hair out about Agnes, who physically pushed others around. She would come up behind people and push them forward or to the side, saying, "Go this way," or, "Come that way."

Unmet Need: *To feel needed and useful*

A member of staff checked into Agnes's past and discovered that she had moved over thirty times during her life as an itinerant worker. She had also lived and worked for a number of years on a ranch. With this knowledge, it became quite obvious that Agnes was mimicking "herding the cattle" and recreating a time when she felt needed and useful.

Solution

The facility obtained a basket on wheels to hold clothing that Agnes could push around. Also, staff set up a clothesline so she could hang up wet clothes and take them down when dried. Nowadays, Agnes no longer needs to push people around and instead spends many hours pushing her basket, greeted by "hellos" and "smiles" rather than the former frowns and angry reactions.

THE DEVASTATING POWER OF DISRESPECT

Richard was still in bed when a staff member came to the door and snapped, "Your breakfast is on the table." Richard was not quite awake but he was hungry and he walked toward the dining room. The same staff member sniped, "You are not allowed to be in the dining room unless you are dressed." Richard turned and yelled in a loud voice, "Get out of my way, you damn witch!" The staff member continued to snipe at Richard and he threatened to hit her. In turn, she reported to her supervisor that Richard was dangerous. His family was told that he had to be relocated to another home.

Unmet Need: *To be treated with respect*

Solution

Richard was moved to another care facility that had staff members who were more tolerant and understanding. Staff members were careful to respect Richard at all times.

THE HAT LADY

Ken and his wife, Lydia, shared a room in the same dementia-specific unit. Ken was known as an easy-going man who usually kept to himself. For her part, Lydia had befriended another lady, Rose, and they spent much time together every day. Ken observed the two women together one afternoon and suddenly shouted an obscenity at Rose and pushed her to the floor. Fortunately, Rose was not injured but she was emotionally upset and terrified of Ken. Lydia was also shaken by the violent episode.

Unmet Need: *To have self-esteem boosted*

In listening carefully to Ken, staff discovered that he had mistakenly believed that the short-haired Rose was a man giving unwelcome attention to his wife. Naturally, he was overcome with anger and emotion at the thought that his place as her husband had been taken by another, robbing him of both his identity and self-esteem.

Solution

The dilemma for the staff was that Lydia loved sharing her room with Rose so the decision was made not to separate the two. Instead, staff devised a very innovative solution to make Rose appear more like a woman. Now—as part of her morning ritual—she selects a beautiful, feminine hat to wear. She has seven hats to choose from; one for each day of the week. Lydia and Rose are happy, the staff is happy, and Ken is happy, too. He never kicked or punched Rose again.

HELP ME! HELP ME!

Every day Norm sat in his room on his own, shouting, "Help me! Help me!" and giving everyone around him a hard time. His behavior had been labeled as "attention seeking." As a management strategy, staff members had begun to withdraw. The more they withdrew, the louder he called. He even began bashing his hands on the wooden table next to him and ramming his elbow into the wall. Both staff members and residents became increasingly agitated.

Unmet Need: *To feel loved*

Solution

Consultation took place among all of the staff members to discover who liked Norm the most and had the best rapport with him. Those staff members were then selected to become his preferred caregivers and were encouraged to show him extra kindness. They gave him extra time and brought him special treats (for example, a home-baked cake or special soap). Within a relatively short time, Norm stopped calling out.

THE "SHOWER PROBLEM"

Shirley was known as a "shower problem." No matter what the staff tried, she just refused to be showered. She was also resistive in other ways: she didn't want to eat—the food was too much or too little, or she wanted someone else's food. She resisted medication and always wanted to sit in someone else's chair. She would not go to bed and continually resisted the efforts of staff.

Unmet Need: *To have self-esteem boosted and to feel loved*

Solution

Staff members resolved to change their attitude and stop viewing Shirley as the "shower problem." Instead, they concentrated on boosting her self-esteem with positive comments, such as, "What a beautiful smile you have Shirley" or "What a lovely outfit you are wearing today." Staff routinely complimented her and used a gentle approach when they asked her to do something. For example, they would ask, "What if I give you a hand?" They also provided explanations before giving assistance or beginning any care aspect. Only those staff members with a rapport with Shirley became responsible in attending to her personal care needs. The positive difference is evident now in Shirley's happy humming during shower time.

IT'S ONLY A TOY!

George kept insisting his toy dog was sick. Staff members had been responding by trying to reassure him by saying, "George, you don't need to worry. Your dog is not sick. It is only a toy and therefore cannot feel any pain or discomfort." Or, "George, what if you give the dog to me and I will take it to the vet for you?" George became increasingly agitated and distressed at their remarks and accepted neither reassurance nor explanations.

Unmet Need: *To have self-esteem boosted, to feel needed and useful, and to give and receive love*

A staff member discovered in George's younger days he had started an animal refuge, which was now a highly regarded facility. In his imagination, George was recreating memories of his dogs and his responsibility for their well-being. He had recreated a time when he had an identity and a purpose in his life.

Solution

Staff members decided on a change of strategy. They acknowledged that George's toy dog was important and that there was a reason behind his behavior. Now when he said that his toy dog was sick, they responded genuinely and sincerely, "George, your concern for the dog is absolutely wonderful. I know of no one else who cares so much. I've been looking for someone who could help us look after our cat and birds. Could I ask you to help? Would that be okay?"

Staff members introduced pets to George's everyday life. They also hung bird feeders and placed bird baths that he could fill and clean—daily jobs that needed his care and attention. George's "dog" made a rapid recovery and was not ill again!

ALIVE IN HER EYES

Lilly continually asked for her husband Ron, who had passed away. He was her beloved husband for 58 years and, until his death, had always been by her side, ready to help and support her. Staff had tried telling the truth, saying, "Lilly, Ron is not coming in today—he passed away 4 years ago." Staff tried fibbing and said, "Lilly, Ron has phoned to say he is busy but he will come in later." Lilly's distress increased and she became aggressive.

Unmet Need: To give and receive love

Lilly was lonely and felt unloved. Recreating memories of her husband helped her experience that love and support.

Solution

Staff members learned that neither the truth nor fibs were effective with Lilly. Her husband Ron was still alive in her mind. It was decided that a few staff would be permanently assigned to Lilly and they would make a special effort to treat her as a friend. They found out she enjoyed receiving small gifts, listening to poetry, and singing religious hymns. Lilly responded well to the special attention and rarely asks about her deceased husband. When she asks about him, staff members always give her a hug and say, "You really miss Ron. Tell me about how the two of you met and fell in love." Lilly then recounts the story and staff members encourage her to reminisce. Afterwards, she and the staff member enjoy tea together. Lilly is no longer distressed or lonely.

SELECTED REFERENCES AND RESOURCES

BOOKS

Bell, V., and Troxler, D. (2001). *The Best Friends Staff: Building a Culture of Care in Alzheimer's Programs*. Baltimore: Health Professions Press.

Bell, V., Troxler, D., Cox, T., and Hamon, R. (2005). *The Best Friends Book of Alzheimer's Activities*. Baltimore: Health Professions Press.

Brooker, D. (2007). *Person-Centred Dementia Care: Making Services Better*. London: Jessica Kingsley Publishers.

Davidson, A. (2006). *A Curious Kind of Widow: Loving a Man with Advanced Alzheimer's*. McKinleyville, Calif.: Fithian Press.

Davis, P. (2003). *The Long Goodbye: Memories of My Father*. New York: Knopf.

Davis, R. (1989). *My Journey into Alzheimer's Disease*. Wheaton, IL: Tyndale House Publishers.

Fazio, S., Seman, D., and Stansell, J. (1999). *Rethinking Alzheimer's Care*. Baltimore: Health Professions Press.

Kitwood, T. (1997). *Dementia Reconsidered: The Person Comes First*. Buckingham, Great Britain: The Open University Press.

Koenig Coste, J. (2004). *Learning to Speak Alzheimer's: A Groundbreaking Approach for Everyone Dealing with the Disease*. New York: Houghton Mifflin.

LaBrake, T. (1996). *How to Get Families More Involved in the Nursing Home: Four Programs that Work and Why*. New York: Haworth Press.

Negri, K. (2005). *Mom, Are You Still There? Finding a Pathway to Peace through Alzheimer's*. Wheat Ridge, Co.: Forget-Me-Not Press.

Strauss, C.J. (2002). *Talking to Alzheimer's: Simple Ways to Connect When You Visit with a Family Member or Friend*. Oakland, Calif.: New Harbinger Publications.

Taylor, R. (2007). *Alzheimer's from the Inside Looking Out*. Baltimore: Health Professions Press.

Thomas, W.H. (1996). *Life Worth Living*. Acton, Mass. VanderWyk & Burnham.

Zgola, J.M. (1999). *Care That Works: A Relationship Approach to Persons with Dementia*. Baltimore: The Johns Hopkins University Press.

ORGANIZATIONS

Alzheimer's Association (312-335-8700 or toll free 800-272-3900) or www.alz.org

Alzheimer's Disease Education and Referral Center (800-438-4380) www.nia.nih.gov/alzheimers

Association for Frontotemporal Dementias (267-514-7221 or toll free 866-507-7222) www.ftd-picks.org

Dementia Care Australia (+61 3 9727 2744) www.dementiacareaustralia.com

Lewy Body Dementia Association (404-935-6444 or toll free 800-539-9767) www.lewybodydementia.org

---

AUDIOVISUAL RESOURCES

- *Choice and Challenge: Caring for Aggressive Adults Across Levels of Care Complaints of a Dutiful Daughter*

- *Freedom of Sexual Expression: Dementia and Resident Rights in Long-Term Care Facilities*
- *Great Nursing Assistants: The Resident's Perspective*
- *He's Doing This to Spite Me*
- *More Than A Thousand Tomorrows*
- The **Spark of Life** *Club Program Education kit, including DVD, available through Dementia Care Australia (+61 3 9727 2744) www.dementiacareaustralia.com*
- The **Spark of Life** *Approach to Difficult Behaviour—Educational In-service DVD, available through Dementia Care Australia (+61 3 9727 2744) www.dementiacareaustralia.com*

These videos may be available through your local library that may obtain them through inter-library loan from the Alzheimer's Association. All videos are available through Terra Nova Films. Call 773-881-8491 or toll free 800-779-8491 for rental or purchase, or go to www.terranova.org.

WEB-BASED TRAINING AND EDUCATION

1. Alzheimer's Association. *CARES: A Dementia Caregiving Approach* includes six, one-hour training modules that are geared to direct care workers, particularly nursing assistants. Each module uses text and streaming video that illustrate how to best care for people with dementia living in residential care settings. For a description of the modules, pricing plans, and a free demonstration, go to www.caresprogram.com.
2. Alzheimer's Association. Learning Academy Online Training includes eight modules with text and streaming video on a variety of care topics. For more details, go to: www.alzceu.org.

3. New York City Department for the Aging. Four free online programs on the different stages of Alzheimer's disease. Go to home2.nyc.gov/html/dfta/html/community/training.shtml.

4. The Aged Care Standards and Accreditation Agency Ltd. Demystifying Dementia Training Package. Available for free at www.accreditation.org.au/DemystifyingDementia.

I N D E X